## Praise for *The Antioxidant Save-Your-Life Cookbook*

Nominated for a World Cookbook Award in the Best Health/Nutrition Cookbook category

"If you've ever wondered how you can eat more of these healthful foods without living on plain carrots and tomatoes, this book will show you how....Easy-to-make, very good recipes, and a couple of the breakfasts are delicious enough to serve for dessert." —*New York Daily News*

"These recipes are kitchen-friendly, palate-pleasing, and dining-enhancement culinary experiences....An ardently recommended addition to the kitchen cookbook collection." —*Midwest Book Review*

"The authors whip up healthy breakfasts, lunches, snacks, and cancer-fighting meals...excellent nutrition information. A valuable section on 'What to Stash and What to Trash' and a glossary of antioxidant terms help readers get their own healthy kitchen underway."
—*Publishers Weekly*

"The Kinderlehrers' recommended diet is naturally high in antioxidants [that] stop the production of free radicals....Recipes will look familiar to anyone knowledgeable about macrobiotic diets with their emphasis on whole grains, fresh vegetables, and fresh fruits." —*Booklist*

"A persuasive approach." —*Pittsburgh Post-Gazette*

"Tempting recipes." —*The Jewish Exponent* (Philadelphia, PA)

OTHER NEWMARKET TITLES BY JANE KINDERLEHRER

*The Smart Baking Cookbook*

*The Smart Chicken and Fish Cookbook*

# The
# Antioxidant
# Save-Your-Life
# Cookbook

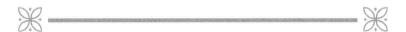

### 150 NUTRITIOUS, HIGH-FIBER, LOW-FAT RECIPES
### TO PROTECT YOU AGAINST THE
### DAMAGING EFFECTS OF FREE RADICALS

Jane Kinderlehrer
and
Daniel A. Kinderlehrer, M.D.

Newmarket Press　New York

*To Harry Kinderlehrer, my lifetime companion, who, though absent, is always present.*
—Jane Kinderlehrer

*To my father, Harry Kinderlehrer, whose love and guidance are always with me.*
—Daniel A. Kinderlehrer, M.D.

First paperback edition June 2007

Paperback ISBN 978-1-55704-760-1

Hardcover ISBN 978-1-55704-301-6

Copyright © 2000 by Jane Kinderlehrer and
Daniel A. Kinderlehrer

This book is published in the United States of America.

1  3  5  7  9  10  8  6  4  2

**Library of Congress Cataloging-in-Publication Data**

Kinderlehrer, Jane.
The antioxidant save-your-life cookbook : 150 nutritious, high-fiber, low-fat recipes to protect you against the damaging effects of free radicals / Jane Kinderlehrer and Daniel A. Kinderlehrer. – 1st ed.
p.    cm.

1. Nutrition.    2. Antioxidants—Health aspects.
3. High-fiber-diet recipes.    4. Low-fat-diet recipes.
I. Title.

RA784.K46        1999

641.5'63—dc21        99-23886

CIP

Quantity Purchases

Companies, professional groups, clubs, and other organizations may qualify for special terms when ordering quantities of this title. For information, write Special Sales Department, Newmarket Press, 18 East 48th Street, New York, NY 10017; call (212) 832-3575; fax (212) 832-3629; or email: info@newmarketpress.com.

www.newmarketpress.com

*Designed by Betty Lew*

Manufactured in the United States of America.

# Contents

# Introduction

## ANTIOXIDANT-SMART EATING AND COOKING

Do you realize that every time you eat the parsley garnish on your plate, you may improve your odds against a whole catalog of devastating illnesses including cancer, cardiovascular disease, osteoporosis, cataracts, and arthritis? How come so many benefits spring from a sprig of parsley? Because parsley, along with many other vegetables and fruits, contains antioxidants—substances that fight the diseases that attack us as we age.

Antioxidants are like guardian angels. They come to the rescue, if they are on hand, and quench the enemy, free radicals, rendering them meek and harmless. Naturally, the fewer free radicals you have to contend with and the more antioxidants you have working for you, the better your chances of good health. Hence the advice to avoid substances that can overwhelm the system, such as cigarette smoke, and to eat plenty of antioxidant-rich foods.

Foremost among the antioxidants are vitamins A, C, and E, carotenoids including beta-carotene (a precursor of vitamin A), and the minerals zinc, selenium, copper, and manganese. These nutrients are found in abundance in vegetables, fruits, and whole grains, which is one reason why it's recommended you eat more of these foods than any other type of food. Nutritionists advise us to eat at least three servings of whole-grain foods each day along with two to four servings of fruits and three to five servings of vegetables. That may sound like a lot of food, but serving sizes are small. One slice of whole wheat bread, or ½ cup of brown rice, equals a serving. Likewise, a small piece of fruit or ½ cup of cooked vegetables counts as one serving. It adds up quickly over the course of a day.

To get the most disease-fighting benefit from vegetables and fruits, rinse them thoroughly to remove pesticide residues before eating. It doesn't matter whether you eat vegetables and fruits raw or cooked. Cooking may destroy some nutrients, but it actually frees up others to work in the body. For best results when cooking vegetables and fruits, however, use only as much water as necessary and steam to a crisp, tender stage to preserve heat- and oxygen-sensitive antioxidants such as vitamin C and carotenoids.

It also makes no difference whether vegetables and fruits are canned, frozen, juiced, or peeled. All forms contain significant amounts of disease-fighting substances. What matters most is eating enough of them. *Supplements won't do the trick.*

Don't look to vitamin and mineral supplements to meet your antioxidant needs. While they may add a little extra to your diet, studies show the real protection comes from nutrients found in foods, not pills. That's likely owing to the combined effects of the many different substances found in foods, some of which we haven't even discovered yet.

For instance, there are more than five hundred carotenoids in foods that go to bat for you against disease. A beta-carotene supplement provides only one type of carotenoid. What's more, recent research not only shows other carotenoids may be even more protective against certain types of cancer, but also we now know beta-carotene supplements may even *increase* health risks for some people.

A diet that contains plenty of beta-carotene-rich foods poses no such risk. And with the hundreds of carotenoids found in deep green or orange-colored foods like spinach, broccoli, winter squash, sweet potatoes, and carrots, you've got a much better chance of building your best defense against disease.

## Variety Is Important

Along with eating a healthy amount of vegetables, fruits, and whole grains, it's also important to eat a variety of them, particularly when it comes to vegetables and fruits. That's because the greatest variety of protective substances may be found in these foods. And it seems as if it takes a variety of substances to adequately guard against the variety of diseases that threaten our health.

Take cancer, for example. Researchers point out that this disease is a multi-step process. To become malignant, a cell must jump through many biochemical hoops. "At almost every one of the steps," says epidemiologist John Potter, M.D., of the University of Minnesota, "there are one or more compounds in vegetables or fruits that will slow up or reverse the process" (*Newsweek,* 25 April 1994).

For instance, limonene found in citrus fruits boosts enzymes that dispose of cancer-causing substances before they have a chance to do their dirty work. And allyl sulfides found in garlic, onions, leeks, and chives help the body produce more of an enzyme that makes it easier to excrete the carcinogens. Other allium substances found in these foods may also interfere with the reproduction of cancer cells. Ellagic acid found in grapes searches out carcinogens and prevents them from making the changes in cell DNA that lead to cancer. Saponins found in soybeans and dried beans may help keep cancer cells from multiplying.

But again, the experts recommend we don't get caught up in eating only certain types of fruits and vegetables for their benefit against a specific disease. Studies conducted worldwide show plant-rich diets in general offer a variety of health advantages, ranging from their content of disease-fighting antioxidants and phytochemicals to their lack of the heart-disease-promoting agents such as saturated fat.

Recently nutritionists have also begun to focus on the value of eating well, not just eating healthfully. That is, we may derive the most health benefits from enjoying our food while we provide our bodies with the many substances food provides to help ensure long and productive lives. I've lived by these principles for many years and have raised four healthy children who are now parents bringing up their own children this way.

I am proud that my youngest son, Dan, has established a career as a medical doctor concerned with holistic health. He has joined me as coauthor of this book, bringing his many years' experience and knowledge to these pages. Included in this work are not only 150 recipes time-tested by both our families but also an excellent piece by Dan on free radicals and life-saving antioxidants, which I know you'll find valuable in understanding the scientific aspects of these components along with the many benefits of the ingredients found here. We hope you use these recipes to help ensure good health for you and your family. We know that they have for ours.

—Jane Kinderlehrer

# Free Radicals and Life-Saving Antioxidants

When I was in college, a free radical was the hothead individual who incited the masses and destabilized the old guard. Now that I am a doctor, the association has shifted, but the theme remains the same.

In medicine, a free radical is a molecule with a single electron in its outer orbit. Highly charged and unstable, it avidly seeks out other molecules with electrons it can steal. In this process, called oxidation, the electron that was robbed of its mate becomes unpaired, and repeats the felony. Unless checked, one free radical can generate hundreds of additional free-radical reactions, causing a string of damaged cells that can lead to aging, cataracts, heart disease, cancer, and immune disorders.

We are, in fact, loaded with free radicals. The act of burning oxygen for energy produces free radicals. Our livers generate free radicals in the processing of metabolic wastes and drugs. When our immune system attacks viruses or bacteria, we utilize free radicals to disarm and destroy the invaders.

We also generate free radicals when we do not particularly want to. Trauma, infection, and aging all result in free radical production that contribute to inflammation and cellular disruption. As well, there are many outside sources to these highly charged molecules—environmental pollutants, cigarette smoke, exhaust fumes, pesticides, herbicides, ozone, ionizing radiation, as well as heavy metals such as mercury, cadmium, lead, and even iron.

As you can see, free radicals are dangerous but not always a bad thing. Free radical production is part of our normal metabolism. Our bodies actually utilize these highly charged, unstable molecules to perform necessary activities, such as the elimination of waste products and killing germs. The danger is when free radical production goes unchecked. For this, mother nature created antioxidants.

When Linus Pauling was fifty-seven, he was diagnosed with prostate cancer. The two-time Nobel Prize winner theorized that he could stabilize the malignant process if he saturated his prostate gland with the antioxidant vitamin C. Generally speaking, prostate cancer that begins at such an early age is highly aggressive and has claimed the lives of men in their relative youth. Pauling, however, survived with all faculties intact into the ripe old age of ninety-three. In the process, he and his wife went year after year without succumbing to the common cold!

Antioxidants are free radical quenchers. They include vitamins A, C, and E; carotenoids, including beta-carotene (a plant precursor of vitamin A); and the minerals zinc, selenium, copper, and manganese. Remember that free radicals are highly reactive because the single unpaired electron desperately seeks a mate. The antioxidants offer themselves in self-sacrifice. They donate an electron, quenching the thirst of the highly charged and destructive free radical. Antioxidants also can stop free radicals from forming in the first place.

Naturally, the fewer free radicals you have to contend with and the more antioxidants you have working for you, the better your chances of good health. Hence, the advice to avoid cigarettes and pollution and to eat plenty of antioxidant-rich foods.

But if you think that this is just microscopic Trivial Pursuit, consider this. Despite enormous gains in the treatment of heart disease, it is still the number one killer in the United States. The process we know as atherosclerotic cardiovascular disease begins as an inflammatory reaction in the walls of the arteries. Antioxidants serve to protect and stabilize the cell membranes of the arterial walls, rendering them less prone to damage when accosted by free radicals in cigarette smoke or oxidized cholesterol.

Many people—and doctors—do not realize that cholesterol is quite benign when compared to oxidatively modified cholesterol. It is the latter molecule, already altered by a free radical encounter, that gets under the skin of the arterial wall and initiates the process we know as atherosclerosis.

Vitamin E is the major antioxidant that protects our membranes. There are a number of studies that demonstrate its role protecting cholesterol from oxidation. When combined with other antioxidants, including vitamin C, beta-carotene, and selenium, its effect is even stronger.

Not surprisingly, there are quite a few epidemiologic studies that document the benefits of vitamin E and other antioxidants in the reduction of heart disease, angina, and cardiovascular mortality. In one well-known Harvard study, a group of 39,910 male health professionals took vitamin E supplements in doses of at least 100 IU daily for a minimum of two years. They had a 30 percent lower relative risk of coronary heart disease compared to men who did not take vitamin E supplements.

Ever hear of "the French paradox"? Frenchmen have a relatively low rate of heart disease despite a high-fat diet, replete with cream sauces and croissants. Investigators believe that the secret lies in the intake of wine, which contains high amounts of proanthocyanidins. These compounds, which belong to the flavonoid family, are found in bilberry, cranberry, black currants, green tea, black tea, grape juice, and wine. They are also available as supplements, derived from pine bark or grape seeds. The main functions of proanthocyanidins are as antioxidants, and they serve to stabilize the walls of our blood vessels.

Many factors interplay in the development of cancer. It has been estimated that 80 to 90 percent of all cancer is environmentally induced, and approximately 35 percent, or over one-third, by diet. Not surprisingly, free radicals play a major role in the process of cancer initiation as well as cancer promotion. Numerous investigations have demonstrated that antioxidants can decrease cancer risk.

Hundreds of studies have now demonstrated that the lower the level of antioxidants in the diet, particularly carotene, vitamin E, and selenium, the higher the likelihood of developing cancer. Epidemiologic studies have demonstrated this association in cancers of the lung, larynx, bladder, esophagus, stomach, colon, prostate, cervix, thyroid, mouth, and throat, as well as leukemia and lymphoma.

Antioxidants help protect against other conditions as well, including aging, Alzheimer's, immune disorders, arthritis, diabetic complications, and eye difficulties, including macular degeneration and cataracts. Studies suggest that these nutrients work best as a team. Vitamins C and E, selenium, and carotene all assist each other in their important roles. There is evidence that beta-carotene, by itself, may not be beneficial. On the other hand, there are over five hundred carotenoids that go to bat for you when you eat the whole food.

In other words, do not look to vitamin and mineral supplements to meet all your antioxidant needs. I recommend a high intake of whole grains, vegetables, and fruits because of the mix of antioxidants and other phytochemicals (plant chemicals) that perform their own magic to stop diseases before they develop.

Tomatoes, for example, contain lycopenes, an antioxidant that protects DNA from toxic damage. A recent study has demonstrated that individuals who have higher amounts of tomatoes and tomato sauce in their diet have a lower risk of cancer. Other citrus fruit contains limonene, which boosts enzymes that dispose of cancer-causing substances, thus helping to prevent cancer. Green tea contains polyphenols, another potent antioxidant, as well as catechins, which help the liver to rid the body of toxins.

Clearly, we need to eat a variety of vegetables, fruits, and whole grains to adequately guard against the variety of diseases that threaten our health. There is some evidence pointing out that certain foods act as better cancer fighters than others. Studies suggest that carrots and green, leafy vegetables appear to wage the good battle against lung cancer, while cruciferous vegetables fight against colon cancer. Fruit appears to be especially effective against cancers of the mouth and neck area, including esophageal cancer. Lettuce and onions help prevent stomach cancer from developing.

Deeply colored vegetables and fruits generally contain more of the important nutrients than their paler cousins. For example, romaine lettuce is a much better source of carotene than iceberg lettuce. Many would argue it tastes better too, adding another good reason for choosing romaine more frequently. Clearly, your best bet is to choose plenty of whole-grain foods, vegetables, and fruits.

As the primary detoxifying organ of the body, the liver has a particularly critical role in the prevention of chronic degenerative diseases, such as cancer, heart disease, and arthritis. Living in the twentieth century, with its added exposures to drugs and environmental pollutants, has added quite a burden to our livers' job description. Luckily, several other natural foods are ready to help out.

Garlics, onions, leeks, and chives contain allyl sulfides, which help regulate phase one liver enzymes and increase the excretion of carcinogens. Cruciferous vegetables, including broccoli, Brussels sprouts, cabbage, cauliflower, collards, kale, kohlrabi, turnips, rutabaga, and mustard greens contain sulforaphane. These compounds boost the production of phase two enzymes, further carting off the dangerous residues that phase one enzymes leave behind. Another constituent of these vegetables, called indoles, stimulates enzymes that decrease estrogen activity and may reduce the risk of breast cancer.

Soybeans are a miracle food because of their action on so many fronts. Soy is replete with isoflavones, primarily genistein and diadzein. These are both antioxidants and phytoestrogens. Phytoestrogens have weak estrogen activity, blocking the effect of natural estrogen and reducing risk of cancer of the breast and prostate. These same chemicals successfully benefit other menopausal problems, including osteoporosis and hot flashes.

There are proteins in soy that suppress the production of enzymes in cancer cells and may slow tumor growth. Soy protein can also decrease cholesterol and the risk of heart disease. Saponins, found in soybeans and dried beans, interfere with DNA production and inhibit tumor growth. In Eastern cultures where soy is the primary dietary protein, the incidence of osteoporosis, heart disease, and cancer are all significantly less than in the United States.

When I was in internal medicine training, I spent most of my time taking care of very sick poeple in the intensive and coronary units. While we did our best to stabilize them, in general their illnesses were too far advanced to cure anyone. It became apparent to me that prevention is the way to go. Our chances of helping people are much greater if we can prevent something before it starts, rather than playing catch-up after it gets going.

In this case, the ounce of prevention is a good healthy diet, and is far superior to a pound of drugs, surgery, or chemotherapy. We have the tools now to provide health insurance for you and your family, which will have far-reaching benefits throughout your lives.

The recipes in the *Save-Your-Life Cookbook* offer a varied feast of antioxidant- and phytochemical-rich dishes to help meet your nutritional needs every day. They will help you take the leap from reading and thinking about good nutrition to actually instituting it. Along with regular exercise and a healthy attitude, it is the best health insurance on the market.

—Daniel A. Kinderlehrer, M.D.

# What to Stash and What to Trash

Start your *Save-Your-Life* antioxidant adventure by discarding negative foods and stocking up on health-building foods.

## WHAT TO STASH

In your good nutrition department, you should have the following foods.

### Wheat Germ, Raw or Toasted

Keep it in the refrigerator or freezer. Raw wheat germ has more nutrients than the toasted because it has not been subjected to heat. The toasted has better keeping quality and a flavor more acceptable to some palates. To give raw wheat germ a toasty flavor, toast about ½ cup in a 250°F oven until light brown and add to the rest in the jar. The whole jar of wheat germ will taste toasted.

Wheat germ is a nutritional gold mine. It provides a lot of protein to repair and rebuild your cells, organs, and tissues; generous amounts of vitamin E to protect you from incipient malignancies; and practically every member of the vitamin B complex in generous amounts. These vitamins are crucial to maintaining a healthy heart, the ability to cope, a lovely complexion, a pleasant disposition, and a clear-thinking mind.

Wheat germ provides a lot of iron, the organic kind that does not fight with vitamin E. Inorganic iron cancels out vitamin E. If you are taking an inorganic iron supplement on a doctor's prescription, make sure you take vitamin E twelve hours later. When Dr. Wilbur Shute treated heart patients with vitamin E, he forbade them to use commercial bread that was fortified with inorganic iron.

## Bran

Coarse miller's bran is available at health food stores and can be added, as a source of additional fiber, to cereals and baked goods. Be sure to increase your liquid intake when you eat bran. Like wheat germ, bran should be kept refrigerated or frozen.

## Whole Wheat Flour

Preferably stone ground. Keep refrigerated or frozen and buy from a source where it is kept refrigerated. Always warm your refrigerated flour before combining it with yeast. Place as much as you need in a 200°F oven for 15 minutes.

## Soy Flour

A protein booster and an important cancer inhibitor: ¼ cup combined with ¾ cup whole wheat flour will greatly enhance the protein and protective value of your baked goods.

## Carob Powder

Carob, which is derived from the pod of the carob tree, is often used as a substitute for chocolate, and many people find the tastes similar. But, unlike chocolate, carob is naturally sweet, thus requiring fewer added sweeteners, and is far less caloric. In the fiber department, carob is in the same league as bran, and its pectin content helps drive down your cholesterol.

Until your family becomes accustomed to the slightly different taste and aroma of carob, add 1 or 2 tablespoons of cocoa to the carob container. The whole thing will taste and smell like cocoa.

## Pressed Oils

Use sunflower, sesame, safflower, corn, canola, or olive oil. Do not use cottonseed oil. Since cotton is not a food, its production is not regulated by safety precautions on the use of pesticides that govern food crops. It is heavily sprayed and who knows how much of this poisonous stuff gets into the oil?

We suggest also that you avoid solvent-expressed oils Some of the solvent, usually hexane, may seep into the oil. Pressed oils are available at natural food stores. Keep them refrigerated.

## Seeds for Eating

Use sesame, sunflower, pumpkin, and poppy seeds. Every seed contains that mysterious vitality that can produce a new plant. Seeds are nature's storehouse of enzymes, vitamins, minerals, protein, and unsaturated fatty acids so essential to the vitality of every cell in your body. Buy them raw and unsalted. Sprinkle them on salads and use them in your baked goods—cookies, cakes, quick breads, kugels, or for noshing.

## Seeds for Sprouting

Discover sprouts, the organic wonder food, and enjoy an explosion of *Save-Your-Life Antioxidants.*

*Consider:* Broccoli has been hailed as the star of the anticancer vegetable kingdom. When broccoli seeds are sprouted those antioxidant values sky-rocket. Broccoli sprouts have been shown to provide sometimes ten times more and sometimes as much as fifty times more than the broccoli.

While similar experiments on other vegetables have not yet been publicized, it is logical to assume that their values, too, will increase when they are sprouted.

Try alfalfa, mung, lentil, wheat, rye, triticale, sesame, and sunflower seeds and raw peanuts, garbanzo beans, and soybeans. They all sprout deliciously and bless you with fantastic nutrients. Get your seeds from food stores, not from garden suppliers where seeds are frequently treated with fungicides.

## Lecithin Granules

Lecithin is a natural emulsifier. By helping to keep cholesterol circulating happily, it helps to prevent the formation of clots in the arteries, thus giving you much better odds against atherosclerosis. Recent research reveals that lecithin increases by a factor of three the amount of cholesterol that can be dissolved in bile salts, the vehicle by which the body rids itself of excess cholesterol.

MIT scientists have determined that lecithin in the diet improves memory and can actually make one "smarter" by manufacturing acetylcholine, which helps the brain to transmit nerve signals.

Because lecithin is high in phosphorous, more calcium is needed to keep the proper balance. Sesame seeds, dry milk powder, green leafy vegetables, and the bones found in canned salmon and sardines are good sources of calcium.

### Beans, Beans, Beans

Use all kinds, especially soybeans. Most beans require presoaking. Exceptions are lentils, split peas, and mung beans. If you keep a tray of soybeans in water in your freezer, you will always have presoaked beans ready to go into your soup, stew, or casseroles. Unlike most beans, soybeans are not starchy. Because of their high protein content, they may be served occasionally as a substitute for meat or eggs. Serve them with a grain, like brown rice or bulgur, and you will enjoy a biologically complete protein.

### Grains

Buckwheat, millet, whole barley, brown rice, bulgur or cracked wheat, and oats are all good sources of nutrients and fiber, which when combined with beans provide a complete protein. (Vegetarians, take note.)

### Molasses

Get the kind that is unsulphured, preferably blackstrap. Use it as a sweetener occasionally instead of honey, or half-and-half with honey, until your family gets accustomed to its rather strong taste. It's a terrific source of iron, and a good source of calcium, potassium, and B vitamins. Put a teaspoon in a cup of hot water for a caffeine-free "coffee" that gives you a lift and no letdown.

### Arrowroot Powder

This natural thickening agent, a source of protein and trace minerals, is derived from the roots of plants that pull minerals from the soil. It is a much more natural and nutritious food than cornstarch, which is highly processed.

### Baking Powder

Buy the kind that is aluminum and sodium free. You'll find it at natural food stores or make your own. To make your own baking powder, combine ¼ teaspoon baking soda with ½ teaspoon cream of tartar. This will give you the rising action of 1 teaspoon commercial baking powder.

——— •◆• ———

## WHAT TO TRASH

### Refined Sugar

British physician John Yudkin says in his book *Sweet and Dangerous,* "Avoid sugar and you will lessen your chances of getting diabetes, dental decay, atherosclerosis, some forms of cancer, obesity, and gout. You will increase your life span and your chances of enjoying a healthy old age."

Scorning the sugar bowl does not mean embracing artificial sweeteners. Many studies reveal that saccharin, for instance, may contribute to cancer formation.

Sugar gives you a rush of energy and then a slide into fatigue and despair. The sugar rushes into your bloodstream without even stopping to make a courtesy call on your liver, which would dole it out slowly.

Once in the bloodstream, it raises your body's blood sugar levels, making you feel high and energetic. But this much sugar in your blood is dangerous, so the insulin comes running out of the Isles of Langerhans in your pancreas and takes that sugar out of your blood; it then deposits it in your cells, where it is stored as fat. But the insulin goes in for overkill. It takes practically all the sugar out of your blood, and there you are in a dark blue funk, feeling more tired and depressed than before, and what do you do? You go scrounging around for a candy bar or a cup of coffee and start the whole vicious cycle over again.

So, if you want to live to be 120 in good health, throw away the sugar bowl and the artificial sweeteners. You can live the sweet life without either.

## Bleached White Flour

A whole book could be written about the crimes of white flour against humanity. Here's only what you need to know to justify a quick switch to whole grains.

The bleaching chemicals destroy vitamin E. Even if the flour is unbleached, it has been deprived of wheat germ, which is the source of vitamin E.

Just think, in the year 1900, before we reaped the consequences of the milling process started in the 1890s, which extracted the vitamin E from the flour, coronary thrombosis was practically unknown. In his book on heart disease, Dr. Paul Dudley White says, "When I graduated from medical school in 1911, I had never heard of coronary thrombosis, which is one of the chief threats to life in the United States and Canada today—an astonishing development in one's own lifetime!" What a terrible price to pay for white flour, foam rubber bread, and emasculated cereals!

## Hydrogenated Fats

Hydrogenation is a process that destroys the original oil with all its mineral compounds and regenerates a new one synthetically. The new one is purified, deodorized, bleached, and an insult to your body. It is believed that these fats pass into the bloodstream from the digestive tract but will not be taken up by the cells of the body, which recognize them as fake. They are probably the main factor creating sludge which may block the blood vessels with tragic results.

Manufacturers use hydrogenated fats in many processed foods, not only in margarine. They're used in peanut butter, mayonnaise, and in practically all prepared cake mixes. Why? Because when these foods are hydrogenated, they do not spoil.

One of the rules you must heed to preserve your family's health is this: *Never buy anything that does not spoil.* Use it before it does. Anything that does not spoil has been embalmed.

— •◆• —

## METRIC CONVERSION CHART

1 teaspoon = 5 ml

1 tablespoon = 15 ml

1 ounce = 30 ml

1 cup = 240 ml/.24 l

1 quart = 950 ml/.95 l

1 gallon = 3.80 l

1 ounce = 28 gr

1 pound = 454 gr/.454 kg

| F.° | 200 | 225 | 250 | 275 | 300 | 325 | 350 | 375 | 400 | 425 | 450 |
|-----|-----|-----|-----|-----|-----|-----|-----|-----|-----|-----|-----|
| C.° | 93 | 107 | 121 | 135 | 149 | 163 | 177 | 191 | 204 | 218 | 232 |

# The
# Antioxidant
# Save-Your-Life
# Cookbook

# Jump Starts: Breakfast

Your morning meal can provide a battalion of antioxidants that scan your body for incipient cancers and jump-start the action that destroys them. Breakfast can certainly be your ally in the fight to live in good health.

It's a good idea to make it a regular morning practice to put on the table a plate of cut-up oranges, with the pith left on and only the outer rind removed. Everyone digs in while assembling breakfast or while waiting to be served.

It's also a good idea to prepare a bowl of fresh fruit salad in the evening, then cover and refrigerate overnight. Topped with yogurt or cottage cheese and some oat bran or wheat germ and some sunflower seeds or granola, you've got a great antioxidant-rich rush-hour breakfast.

The orange rind, usually discarded, provides very important antioxidants. The inner white rind is a source of valuable bioflavonoids that, in partnership with vitamin C, provide valiant protective service for body and soul. All of the recipes suggested for breakfast, from instant milk shakes to luscious pancakes, will provide many valuable antioxidants.

## ENJOY AN APPLE A DAY AND START WITH BREAKFAST

Red and Golden Delicious, Winesap, Jonathan, Stayman, Granny Smith, Macintosh—what a world of juicy flavor their names imply!

And yes, it's true. An apple a day may keep the doctor away. Apples provide an appreciable amount of vitamins C, B₁, B₂, pantothenic acid, and small quantities of antioxidant vitamins E, B₆, and carotene. The apple further enriches our bodies with a good supply of important minerals—calcium, phosphorus, iron, iodine, a small amount of sodium, and a large amount of potassium. Magnesium, manganese, and zinc are also represented.

Besides delighting our taste buds with their juicy succulence, perhaps the apple's most important contribution to health lies in its rich supply of pectin, a soluble fiber that has been found to lower cholesterol levels. Some of the pectin is found in the pulp, but it is also present in appreciable quantities in the pit, skin, and core of the apple.

Keep an apple handy in your handbag or briefcase. Keep a bag of them in your car. Stuck in a traffic jam? Make it a pause that refreshes. Bite into an apple.

Apples are a good aid to helping you lose weight naturally. They are low in fat. The result is a sweet, tart package, naturally rich in vitamins and minerals, that satisfies while supplying relatively few calories.

It's a good idea to consume some apples raw and some cooked for a diversity of available nutrients and other valuable substances. Enjoy the versatility, flavor, and nutrients of apples in these recipes.

• ◆ •

# Apple Frittata

An Italian-style omelet, great for brunch, lunch, or supper.

> 1 teaspoon butter or olive or canola oil
> 1 large apple (preferably Golden Delicious), halved, cored, and coarsely
>   chopped
> 4 eggs, beaten
> Pepper to taste

Melt butter in skillet over medium heat. Add the apple and cook 1 to 2 minutes, until golden. Pour in eggs. Sprinkle with a pinch of pepper. Cook over high heat until bottom is lightly browned and eggs are almost set. Turn and cook a minute or so longer, or until eggs are light and fluffy.

*Yield:* 3 servings

---

**Each serving provides approximately 148 calories., 9 g protein, 3.5 g saturated fat, 4.2 g unsaturated fat, 80 mg sodium.**

---

# Sprout Omelet with Tomatoes

A battery-charging breakfast, lunch, or light supper rich in protective nutrients: Selenium provided by the eggs brings you some protection from cardiovascular disease as well as cancer. Tomatoes contain lycopene, a valuable antioxidant that has been shown to reduce the chances of lung and prostate cancers.

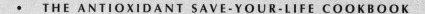

4 eggs, beaten

3 tablespoons milk

2 green onions, chopped

1 tablespoon chopped fresh dill, or
   your favorite herb

1 teaspoon canola oil

1 teaspoon butter

1 medium tomato, coarsely
   chopped

½ cup sunflower seed sprouts

½ cup alfalfa sprouts

In a bowl, combine eggs, milk, onions, and the herbs, and mix well. In a skillet over medium heat combine the oil and butter and heat, add egg mixture and cook until mixture begins to set. Add the tomato and sprouts. Using a spatula fold the omelet over, slide it onto a warm plate, and top with alfalfa sprouts.

*Yield:* 4 servings

---

**Each serving provides approximately 130 calories, 8.5 g protein, 2.8 g saturated fat, 6 g unsaturated fat, 60 mg sodium.**

---

# Granola

A powerhouse of antioxidants to brighten your day and your life. This granola is made with wheat germ and sunflower seeds for vitamin E, dried apricots and shredded carrots for beta-carotene, and grated orange rind for the valuable antioxidants in orange skin oil. The soy component provides genistein, which may help nip cancer cells in the bud. They also help you to feel well fed on fewer calories, and the popcorn adds fiber and crunch and very few calories.

½ cup raisins

½ cup chopped apricots

½ cup rolled oats

½ cup sunflower seeds

¼ cup sesame seeds

¼ cup chopped almonds

½ cup wheat germ

½ cup soy nuts

2 cups popped whole corn

1 teaspoon cinnamon

1 tablespoon grated orange rind

1 medium carrot, pared and
   shredded

Soak the raisins and apricots in ½ cup water for 2 hours or overnight, or microwave for 1 minute on full power.

Preheat oven to 250°F.

In a large mixing bowl, combine the rest of the dry ingredients with the orange rind and the carrot and toss.

Spread the mixture in a thin layer on a cookie sheet lined with parchment paper or sprayed with nonstick cooking spray. Bake for 20 minutes, or until the mixture is dry and crunchy. Stir in the raisins and apricots and bake 5 more minutes.

## MICROWAVE METHOD

Microcook water, raisins, and apricots on high for 1 minute. In a large mixing bowl, combine the rest of the dry ingredients with the orange rind and carrot and toss. Spread half of the moistened mixture in a microwave-safe dish about 12 by 9 inches and microcook, uncovered, on medium power for 5 minutes. Add the raisin and apricot mixture and microcook 1 minute more, stirring several times during cooking. Place in the oven for about 5 minutes, or until thoroughly dried out. Repeat the procedure with the other half of the mixture.

*Yield:* About 2 quarts

---

**Each ¹/₂-cup serving provides approximately 80 calories, 3 g protein, 1 g saturated fat, 6 g unsaturated fat.**

---

### GRATED ORANGE RIND

If you are accustomed to starting the day with a glass of orange juice, you may want to switch to a whole orange. You will be getting more antioxidants from the flavonoids in the pulp; you will be getting valuable fiber too. The oil in the orange skin is also a valuable antioxidant. Dried and grated, it gives life to all manner of breakfast treats.

Scrub the orange, dry it, then, with a vegetable peeler, peel the top skin, the orange part. Let it dry, on a radiator, in a dehydrator, or simply exposed to the air. Then grind it into a fine crumb or powder in a food mill or coffee grinder or with a rolling pin. Place in a small jar and use it to pep up your morning cereal, in muffins, cookies, cakes, rice puddings, and just about everything you bake.

# Buckwheat Cereal

Replenish your energy and give your blood an injection of vitamin E and other antioxidants with a steaming bowl of buckwheat for breakfast. Unlike other cereals, buckwheat is rich in vitamin E and the whole family of B vitamins, and has twice as much hard-working calcium as other grains. Buckwheat is a distinguished member of the rhubarb family and not a true grain and can therefore be enjoyed by those who are allergic to grains.

1 cup buckwheat groats
2 cups water
¼ teaspoon kelp, salt, or vegetable seasoning

Sprinkle the buckwheat into boiling water. Stir for 1 minute. Reduce heat to simmer, cover the pot, and cook for about 10 minutes.

Serve with yogurt, or milk and fruit, and a bit of honey or strawberry jam.

*Yield:* 4 servings

## MICROWAVE METHOD

In a 4-cup measure, combine 1 cup buckweat groats and 2 cups of water. Stir. Micro-cook on high for 5 minutes.

---

**Each serving, without topping, provides approximately 81 calories, 3 g protein, 6 g fat.**

---

# Hot Apple Grape-Nuts Crunch

A delicious, body-warming cereal enriched with soy, which provides the cancer fighter genistein; oats for vitamin E and fiber; vitamin A, which provides a measure of protection from stroke; and walnuts for essential fatty acids that lower cholesterol, reduce inflammation, and provide lovely crunch and flavor. Try it, you'll love it.

¼ cup rolled oats
¼ cup soy flakes
¼ cup Grape-Nuts cereal
⅔ cup apple juice

1 apple, chopped
2 tablespoons raisins or currants
Pinch of cinnamon

Combine all of the ingredients in a 1-quart saucepan. Bring to a boil, lower heat, and simmer, stirring for 1 minute.

## MICROWAVE METHOD

Combine ingredients in a microsafe bowl and microcook on medium for 1 minute.

*Yield:* 2 servings

---

**Each serving provides approximately 160 calories, 2.4 g protein, 1 g unsaturated fat.**

---

# Oatmeal Cookie Crunch Cereal

Though this dish has no added sweetener, it has a delicious sweetness that everyone in my family loves. The raisins sweeten the water in which the oats and soy flakes are cooked. The nuts and seeds give it crunch and are full of antiaging, anticancer antioxidants. The sunflower seeds provide vitamin E, the Brazil nuts provide selenium, which works in concert with vitamin E to neutralize damage from free radicals and help you stay young longer.

| | |
|---|---|
| 2 cups water | ½ teaspoon cinnamon |
| ½ cup raisins | ½ teaspoon vanilla |
| ½ cup rolled oats | ¼ cup sunflower seeds |
| ½ cup soy flakes | ¼ cup chopped walnuts |
| 2 tablespoons oat bran | 2 Brazil nuts, chopped |

In a 1-quart saucepan, combine 2 cups of water and the raisins. Bring to a boil. Add oats gradually, stirring. Add soy flakes, oat bran, cinnamon, and vanilla. Reduce heat and cook for about 8 minutes. Ladle into bowls and top with seeds and nuts. Serve with milk or yogurt.

*Note:* The uneaten oatmeal can be frozen up to two weeks in single-portion containers. When you want to microwave a quick breakfast, you've got it made.

## MICROWAVE METHOD

In a 2-quart casserole, combine all ingredients. Mix well. Microcook on high for 4 or 5 minutes; stir, then cook 4 or 5 minutes more, depending on consistency desired.

*Yield:* 4 servings

---

**Each serving provides approximately 188 calories, 5.6 g protein, 1.7 g saturated fat, 4.5 g unsaturated fat, 3 mg sodium.**

---

# Feather-Light Pancakes

These delicious pancakes provide the cancer-fighting genistein of the soy and selenium of the eggs; and the protein, vitamin A, and potassium of the yogurt. I love to serve these with prune and apricot whip.

2 eggs
1½ cups plain nonfat yogurt
1 tablespoon softened butter or
   olive oil
1 cup whole wheat flour

¼ cup soy flour
2 tablespoons wheat or oat bran
1 teaspoon baking powder
½ teaspoon baking soda

Combine all ingredients in blender or food processor and process only until batter is smooth. Lightly oil a hot griddle or skillet. Pour about ¼ cup of batter for each griddle cake. When they get bubbly, turn them over and cook for about 2 minutes.

*Yield:* About 20 pancakes

---

**Each pancake provides approximately 47 calories, 6 g protein, .3 g saturated fat, .4 g unsaturated fat, 1.2 mg sodium.**

---

# Prune and Apricot Whip

Great on pancakes, but also delicious spread on toast, a bagel, or a muffin. It also makes a lovely dessert when served in stemmed glasses and topped with sunflower seeds. Apricots are packed with beta-carotene, which some studies have shown to cut the risk of lung cancer in half. The combination of apricots and prunes is potent ammunition against constipation and cancer. This is one of those toppings that seems too good to be good for you.

8 pitted prunes
8 dried apricots
¼ cup plain yogurt

In a small bowl, soak the prunes and apricots in water or fruit juice to cover, for an hour or overnight. When the fruit is softened, drain and puree in a blender or food processor until smooth. Add the yogurt and blend until smooth.

*Yield:* ³/₄ cup

---

**Each 2 tablespoons provides approximately 33 calories.**

---

# Zucchini Cheese Pancakes

Zucchini, a member of the squash family, is a storehouse of phytochemicals. Serve these scrumptious pancakes with tomato sauce for double-duty anticancer insurance. The phytochemicals in tomatoes snuff out the formation of cancer-causing substances before they do their dirty work, while the garlic and onions deliver valuable allium compounds.

| | |
|---|---|
| 3½ cups grated zucchini | ¼ cup soy flour |
| ⅓ cup grated onion | ¼ cup oat bran |
| 1 clove garlic, minced | ¼ cup wheat germ |
| ⅔ cup grated Parmesan cheese | 2 tablespoons lecithin granules |
| 4 eggs, lightly beaten | ½ teaspoon oregano |
| ¼ cup whole wheat pastry flour | ½ teaspoon thyme |

In a large bowl, combine zucchini, onion, garlic, and cheese. Mix in the eggs, then the flours, oat bran, wheat germ, lecithin, oregano, and thyme.

Pour ¼ cup of batter for each pancake onto a hot, buttered skillet or griddle and flatten with a wooden spoon. Cook about 3 minutes or until brown, turn, using a spatula, and brown on the other side.

*Yield:* 32 pancakes

Each pancake provides approximately 40 calories, 2.8 g protein, 1 g fat.

# Sweet Potato Pancakes

Serve these comforting griddle cakes with maple syrup or applesauce for breakfast or for lunch with mushrooms and sour cream or yogurt.

⅓ cup soy flour

⅓ cup whole wheat pastry flour

2 teaspoons baking powder

2 eggs, lightly beaten

1 cup milk

3 tablespoons honey

2 medium sweet potatoes, unpeeled, scrubbed, grated

2 tablespoons canola, olive, or peanut oil

In a mixing bowl, combine the flours and baking powder.

In another bowl, or in the food processor, whisk together the eggs, milk, and honey.

Add the dry ingredients to the egg mixture. Blend only until batter is evenly moistened. Fold in the sweet potatoes.

In a heavy nonstick skillet over medium heat, heat 1 tablespoon of the oil. Ladle ¼ cup of batter into the skillet. With the back of the ladle, spread batter out to about 6 inches in diameter. Cook for about 1 minute, then, using a spatula, turn and brown the other side. Continue with remaining batter, adding more oil as needed to prevent sticking. Serve immediately or keep warm in a 200°F oven.

*Yield:* About 10 pancakes

---

**Each pancake provides approximately 180 calories, 5.8 g protein, 1.2 g saturated fat, 3.3 g unsaturated fat, 25 mg sodium.**

# Aunt Betty's Oven-Baked Apple Pancake

The fiber in apples lowers cholesterol and it has been shown to reduce the risk of a host of cancers.

2 large eggs

1 cup milk

1 tablespoon honey

1 tablespoon unsalted butter, softened

¼ cup whole wheat pastry flour

¼ cup soy flour or powder

2 tablespoons wheat germ

1 large Golden Delicious apple, halved, cored, and cut into wedges

1 tablespoon Sucanat

¼ teaspoon cinnamon

Preheat oven to 425°F.

Generously spray a 10-inch skillet with nonstick cooking spray.

In a bowl or food processor, whisk together eggs, milk, honey, and butter.

In another bowl, sift together the flours and wheat germ. Combine the two mixtures and blend well.

Core the apple and cut into wedges. In a bowl, toss the apple wedges with Sucanat and the cinnamon.

Pour batter into skillet and arrange apple wedges evenly on top.

Cook for 20 minutes, then reduce temperature to 350°F and cook another 10 minutes, or until pancake is golden, center is set, and the edge is puffed. Serve immediately.

*Yield:* 3 servings

**Each serving provides approximately 283 calories, 11 g protein, 4.4 g saturated fat, 4.2 g unsaturated fat, 71 mg sodium.**

# Pumpkin Pancakes

If the aroma of these pancakes doesn't make your mouth water, the gorgeous hue will. Pumpkin is an excellent source of beta-carotene, which is believed to reduce the risk of certain types of cancer and heart disease. Serve these with maple syrup, applesauce, or yogurt.

½ cup cornmeal

1 cup boiling water

¾ cup milk

¼ cup cooked pumpkin puree

1 cup whole wheat pastry flour

2 teaspoons baking powder

1 tablespoon honey

1 egg, beaten

1 tablespoon olive or canola oil

Add the corn meal to the boiling water, stirring constantly. Add milk, stirring until smooth. Stir in the pumpkin. Add the flour mixed with the baking powder. Stir in the honey, egg, and oil. Ladle onto a greased grill or skillet, and cook until bubbles form on the surface. Turn and continue cooking until the flip side is golden brown.

*Yield:* About 12 pancakes

---

**Each pancake provides approximately 71 calories, 3 g protein, .8 g saturated fat, 2 g unsaturated fat, 16 mg sodium.**

---

# Maple-Walnut Waffles

These are perfect for a leisurely weekend breakfast. Spoon applesauce and a little maple-flavored yogurt on top of each waffle and savor every delicious—and healthy—bite.

Consider: Both whole wheat and wheat germ provide vitamin E, which can help ward off heart attacks and all kinds of cancers. Walnuts are a good source of EFA (essential fatty acids) essential to the very beat of your heart.

½ cup whole wheat pastry flour
½ cup soy flour
2 tablespoons wheat germ
1 tablespoon lecithin granules
1 tablespoon oat bran
2 teaspoons baking soda

1 tablespoon olive or canola oil
1½ cups buttermilk or plain yogurt
1 egg, beaten
1 tablespoon maple syrup
½ cup coarsely chopped walnuts

In a medium-size bowl, combine the flours, wheat germ, lecithin, oat bran, and baking soda.

In a small bowl, blend the oil, buttermilk or yogurt, egg, and maple syrup only until ingredients are combined. Do not beat.

Heat the waffle iron. Brush lightly with oil or butter. Pour in enough batter to just fill—do not overfill. Close and cook until steaming stops and waffles are crisp and golden brown.

*Yield:* Six 4-segment waffles

---

**Each waffle provides approximately 200 calories, 10 g protein, 1 g saturated fat, 10 g unsaturated fat, 66 mg sodium.**

---

# Cheesy Banana Toast

This little treat is delicious, satisfying, and simple to prepare. The cheese provides protein for muscles and calcium for strong bones, the whole-grain bread provides complex carbohydrates, B vitamins for energy, and protective vitamin E. The bananas are loaded with potassium, which is vital for maintaining the proper balance of body fluids.

> ½ cup low-fat cottage cheese
> 2 slices whole-grain toast
> Dash of cinnamon
> Dash of grated orange rind (page 8)
> 1 banana, sliced
> 1 tablespoon sesame seeds

Spread ¼ cup of cottage cheese on each piece of bread. Sprinkle with cinnamon, sesame seeds, and orange rind, and arrange banana slices on top. Toast in a toaster oven or in the broiler until cheese is hot and bread is slightly toasted.

*Yield:* 1 or 2 servings

---

**Each slice provides 168 calories, 13 g protein, .5 g saturated fat, 2 g unsaturated fat, 205 mg sodium.**

---

# Apple and Pear Crêpes with Raspberry Syrup

These elegant crêpes are rich in several powerful disease-fighting substances. They are wonderful for a company brunch, a vegetarian dinner, or a romantic lunch.

Believe it or not, this ambrosial dish is full of antidisease ammunition. The phytochemicals in the soy and the detoxifying acid in the apples, pears, and raspberries have been shown to snuff out the formation of cancer-causing free radicals.

## Crêpes

    3 eggs
    ½ cup soy flour
    ½ cup whole wheat pastry flour
    1 cup water or apple juice

## Syrup

    2 cups fresh or frozen raspberries
    2 tablespoons honey
    ½ teaspoon vanilla
    2 teaspoons arrowroot powder
    ¼ cup water

## Filling

    3 tart apples, thinly sliced
    2 pears, thinly sliced
    2 tablespoons unsalted butter

    1 tablespoon honey
    3 tablespoons raisins
    ½ teaspoon cinnamon

### TO MAKE THE CRÊPES

In a large mixing bowl or food processor, combine eggs, flours, and water or apple juice and mix to make a smooth batter the consistency of light cream. Pour into a 2-cup measure with a pouring lip and refrigerate for at least 30 minutes.

### TO MAKE THE SYRUP

In a small saucepan, combine raspberries, honey, and vanilla. Stir over low heat until just below boiling. Combine arrowroot powder and water, and add to raspberry mixture. Cook over low heat until thickened, about 5 minutes. This results in a jamlike consistency.

## TO MAKE THE FILLING

Sauté apple and pear slices in the butter until slightly softened. Stir in honey, raisins, and cinnamon. Remove from heat and cover to keep warm.

To complete the crêpes, pour ¼ cup of the batter into a nonstick 8-inch skillet or crêpe pan and tilt to spread evenly. Cook for 1 minute on each side. Remove from pan to a towel. Repeat with remaining batter.

Spread about 3 tablespoons of the filling down the center of each crêpe and fold both sides over the filling. Garnish with raspberry syrup, or, if you prefer, plain raspberries.

*Yield:* Makes 16 filled crêpes

---

Each crêpe provides 83 calories, 2 g protein, 2.8 g saturated fat. With topping, each crêpe provides 99 calories, 2.2 g protein, 2.8 g saturated fat.

---

# Cornmeal-Cranberry Muffins

These flavorful muffins provide health insurance on many levels. The cranberries help prevent urinary tract infections. The prune puree offers hefty amounts of iron, potassium, and fiber while the cornmeal is a good source of potassium. Equally important, though, my grandkids love 'em.

¾ cup unsweetened applesauce

⅔ cup buttermilk or plain yogurt

¼ cup honey

1 large egg

2 tablespoons Prune Puree
   (page 158)

1 cup whole wheat pastry flour

½ cup soy flour

¼ cup oat bran

¼ cup lecithin granules

½ cup cornmeal

2 teaspoons baking soda

1 cup cranberries

Preheat oven to 350°F. Place liners in twelve ½-cup muffin cups or lightly coat with nonstick cooking spray.

In mixing bowl or food processor, blend together applesauce, buttermilk or yogurt, honey, egg, and prune puree.

In another bowl, combine the flours, oat bran, lecithin granules, cornmeal, and baking soda; stir dry ingredients into the batter just until moistened. Stir in cranberries; do not overmix. Spoon into muffin cups and bake 20 to 25 minutes.

*Yield:* 12 golden muffins flecked with red

---

Each muffin provides approximately 135 calories, 4 g protein, a mere trace of fat, 161 mg sodium.

# The Best Bran Muffins

These muffins are proof that the road to good health is paved with delicious things.

Packed with carrots, which are rich in antioxidants (which have been shown to lower the risk of developing macular degeneration), the muffins also provide genistein, a phytochemical in the soy family that cuts off the lifeline of tiny tumors, preventing their growth and demolition potential.

The lecithin emulsifies fat, preventing it from forming clots in your arteries.

And that's not all. You're also benefiting from cancer-deterring selenium in the Brazil nuts.

½ cup raisins, plumped
¾ cup milk combined with
  ¾ cup water
1 egg
1 tablespoon canola or olive oil
1 cup millers bran or crushed bran cereal flakes
½ cup whole wheat pastry flour
½ cup soy flour

2 tablespoons oat bran
2 teaspoons baking powder
½ teaspoon baking soda
1 teaspoon cinnamon
½ teaspoon nutmeg
1½ cups grated carrots (about 4 medium to large carrots)
4 Brazil nuts

Plump raisins in a small dish with a little water or fruit juice and microwave for 1 or 2 minutes on high.

In a large bowl, combine all the dry ingredients. In another bowl or in the food processor, blend the milk–water mixture, the egg, and the oil. Combine all the dry ingredients and spices, add them to the wet ingredients, and blend briefly just to combine.

Stir in the carrots and raisins. Grate some Brazil nuts over each muffin.

Preheat oven to 400°F.

Spoon batter into a 12-cup muffin pan lightly greased or spritzed with cooking spray. Bake for 15 minutes and test. If cake tester inserted in the middle of a muffin comes out wet, turn off the oven and let them sit there for another 5 minutes or until cake tester comes out clean.

*Yield:* 12 muffins

---

**Each muffin provides approximately 110 calories, 3 g protein, .9 g saturated fat, 2 g unsaturated fat, 10 mg sodium.**

---

# Apricot, Currant, and Date Oatmeal Muffins

These low-calorie dynamos are antioxidant rich—a real nutrition bargain. They pack well too, and are perfect for a portable breakfast, a lunch box treat, or tucked into a coat pocket for a snack on the road.

¾ cup orange, apple, or pineapple
    juice

⅔ cup buttermilk or plain yogurt

¼ cup honey

1 large egg

1 cup rolled oats

2 tablespoons unsweetened
    applesauce

⅓ cup dried currants

⅓ cup dried apricots that have
    been cut into small pieces

2 tablespoons chopped dates

1 cup whole wheat pastry flour

½ cup soy flour

2 teaspoons baking soda

½ teaspoon orange or lemon zest

2 tablespoons slivered almonds
    (optional garnish)

Preheat oven to 350°F.

Place liners in twelve ½-cup muffin cups or lightly grease or use nonstick cooking spray.

In mixing bowl or food processor, mix the juice, buttermilk or yogurt, honey, and egg. Add the oats, applesauce, and dried fruits.

In another bowl, combine the flours, baking soda, and zest. Stir into the batter just until moistened. Do not overmix. Spoon into muffin cups; garnish with the almonds. Bake 20 to 25 minutes, until deliciously golden.

*Yield:* 12 muffins

---

Each muffin provides approximately 148 calories, 4 g protein, practically no fat, 200 mg sodium.

---

# Four-B Muffins

Bananas, blueberries, bran, and Brazil nuts—a delicious artillery of disease-fighting ingredients. High in fiber and rich in energizing antioxidant nutrients, these muffins will help you keep your sunny side up.

1 cup mashed ripe bananas

¾ cup buttermilk or yogurt

¼ cup honey

1 large egg

2 tablespoons olive or canola oil

½ cup wheat bran

½ cup oat bran

½ cup Grape-Nuts cereal

1 cup whole wheat pastry flour

2 teaspoons baking soda

2 teaspoons cinnamon

1 cup blueberries

4 Brazil nuts, grated or finely
   chopped

Preheat oven to 350°F.

Spritz 12 muffin cups with nonstick cooking spray.

In mixing bowl or food processor blend bananas, buttermilk or yogurt, honey, egg, and oil. Mix in the wheat and oat brans and let stand for 5 minutes.

In another bowl or on a sheet of wax paper, mix the Grape-Nuts, flour, baking soda, and cinnamon. Stir blueberries into the batter. Blend but do not overmix. Spoon into cups. Garnish with grated Brazil nuts. Bake 20 to 25 minutes, until golden.

*Yield:* 12 muffins

---

**Each muffin provides 146 calories, 4 g protein, 1 g saturated fat, 2 g unsaturated fat, 287 mg sodium.**

---

# Carob-Peanut-Banana Breakfast Shake

If you don't have time for a sit-down breakfast, enjoy this refreshing battery charger. It can be whizzed up in seconds.

  1 cup milk
  ¼ cup homemade or natural peanut butter
  1 mellow banana
  1 tablespoon carob powder
  1 tablespoon honey or molasses

In a blender or food processor, combine the ingredients and whiz for about 2 minutes or until thick and frothy. If you have any of the mixture left over, pour it into small paper or plastic cups. Insert wooden sticks or the handle end of a plastic spoon and freeze for a delightful after-school snack.

*Yield:* 2 servings

---

**One serving contains approximately 300 calories, 150 g protein, 7.4 g fat, 60 g sodium.**

---

# Fruity Yogurt Drink

Deliciously refreshing, this drink makes a great breakfast even late wakers have time for and rids you instantly of the hungries. Blueberries offer miraculous help to opposing problems. They help combat diarrhea, yet act as a laxative in some people.

 1 banana
 1 cup plain yogurt
 1 cup chilled orange juice
 1 cup blueberries or hulled strawberries
 ½ teaspoon vanilla
 1 teaspoon honey

Reserve 3 slices of the banana and combine the rest with remaining ingredients in blender or food processor. Process until the mixture is smooth. Pour the mixture into 3 glasses and garnish each one with a banana slice.

*Yield:* 3 luscious drinks

---

**Each serving provides approximately 118 calories, 4 g protein, .5 g saturated fat, .3 g unsaturated fat, 29 mg sodium.**

# APPETIZERS, SIDE DISHES, AND SNACKS

Side dishes give you a chance to sample foods that don't usually occur on your menu. They can be for tasting or consuming. You get a chance to sample and become acquainted with unfamiliar foods. The Japanese maintain that every time you sample a new food, you add seventy-five days to your life.

Be sure to try the Eggplant Caviar, the Sweet Potato Chips, the Stuffed Celery, and all the other intriguing recipes in this chapter. Every one of them offers you a whole menu of antioxidants to enhance your life and help you achieve a multiple of seventy-five days.

# Eggplant Caviar

I have served this dish for many years but never realized before how much potential protection from heart disease and cancer I was getting with every bite. Each of the ingredients provides some kind of protection from free radical and carcinogen damage.

2 medium-size eggplants, about
   1½ pounds, halved lengthwise
¼ cup minced onion
1 teaspoon minced garlic
½ cup finely chopped parsley

1 tablespoon lemon juice
½ cup yogurt
¼ cup finely chopped green
   pepper
2 tablespoons cubed tomato

Microwave the eggplants on high for about 5 minutes or until collapsed. Scrape out the pulp and coarsely chop. Transfer to a bowl and add the remaining ingredients. Mix well and chill. Serve with whole wheat pita cut in triangles and toasted, or with crisp raw vegetables.

*Yield:* About 3 cups, 6 servings

---

**Each serving provides approximately 32 calories, 1 g protein, just a trace of fat, 2 g sodium.**

# Sweet Potato Chips

The healthy antioxidant- and phytochemical-packed alternative to the ubiquitous high fat chip. Noshers will double dip for these and get a double helping of anticancer carotenes.

  1 medium sweet potato or yam, well scrubbed and unpeeled, thinly sliced
  3 tablespoons frozen orange juice concentrate, undiluted
  3 tablespoons soy nuts, crushed
  3 tablespoons sesame seeds
  ½ teaspoon cinnamon

Place the orange juice in a saucer.

Crush the soy nuts and combine with the sesame seeds and cinnamon.

Preheat the oven to 325°F.

Cover an ovenproof tray with foil. Spritz with nonstick cooking spray.

Dip the sweet potato slices in the orange juice and then in the soy nut mixture. Place on the prepared tray.

Bake for 20 to 30 minutes or until chips are crisp and irresistible.

*Yield:* About 30 crisps

---

**Each crisp provides approximately 2 calories.**

---

# Vegetarian Stuffed Cabbage

Cabbage and its cousins in the cruciferous family are a potent antidote to incipient cancers. Highly nutritious, versatile, and inexpensive, cabbage is enjoying a renaissance. It is showing up on menus in top-flight restaurants all over the country. These bite-size rolls pack a powerful punch of anticancer fighters.

| | |
|---|---|
| ¼ cup uncooked brown rice | 1 medium-size tomato, finely |
| ⅓ cup water | chopped |
| 3 tablespoons olive oil | 1 teaspoon dried oregano |
| 1 medium-size onion, finely | ½ tablespoon soy sauce |
| chopped | ¼ cup pine nuts or sunflower seeds |
| 2 tablespoons chopped green | Cayenne pepper to taste |
| pepper | 12 large cabbage leaves |
| 1½ cups sliced mushrooms | 1½ cups tomato sauce |
| 2 cloves garlic, minced | ½ lemon, thinly sliced |
| 1½ teaspoons minced fresh basil, or | Chopped fresh mint or parsley |
| ½ teaspoon dried | |

In a 2-quart saucepan, bring rice and water to a boil. Cover, reduce heat to low, and cook until water has been almost completely absorbed, about 10 minutes.

Add 2 tablespoons of oil, the onion, and green pepper to rice. Cook over low heat, stirring frequently, until vegetables are just limp. Then stir in mushrooms, garlic, basil, tomato, oregano, and soy sauce. Cook gently, uncovered, until liquid from the tomato has been absorbed. Add pine nuts or sunflower seeds and sprinkle with cayenne. Remove pan from heat and set aside.

If cabbage leaves have thick ribs, trim backs of ribs even with the leaves, keeping leaves intact. Steam just until color deepens.

Gently place leaves in a single layer on a clean surface. Place a tablespoon of stuffing at base of each leaf. Fold leaf end over stuffing, fold in sides and roll.

Place the remaining tablespoon of oil in a thin layer over the bottom of a heavy saucepan large enough to hold all the rolls in a single layer. Pour ¾ cup of tomato sauce in the pan, add cabbage rolls, seam-side down, cover with remaining tomato sauce, and simmer, covered, for 45 minutes.

Place lemon slices over cabbage rolls and simmer an additional 20 minutes. Garnish with chopped mint or parsley.

*Yield:* 12 cabbage rolls

---

Each roll provides approximately 53 calories, 2.3 g protein, .5 g saturated fat, 3.7 g unsaturated fat, 64 mg sodium.

---

# Stuffed Celery with Yogurt Cream Cheese and Sunflower Seeds

Celery has been shown to deter the development of stomach cancer; yogurt is antibacterial as well as anticancer; and sunflower seeds are a good source of vitamin E, which, if eaten in early adulthood, seems to block the onset of Parkinson's in late adulthood.

Full of health protectors and low-calorie too, these are the perfect healthy TV snack.

3 stalks of celery
1 cup Yogurt Cream Cheese (recipe follows)
½ cup sunflower seeds

Use celery stalks that are groovy so they can better hold the filling.

Combine the cheese and sunflower seeds and fill the celery grooves. Cut each stalk in 4 pieces.

Refrigerate until serving time.

*Yield:* 12 pieces

---

Each piece provides 20.7 calories, 1 g protein, .3 g saturated fat, 1 g unsaturated fat, 1.8 mg sodium.

---

### Yogurt Cream Cheese

Place a pint of plain yogurt in a colander lined with three layers of cheesecloth or a clean tea towel. Let it drain into a bowl for several hours, or overnight. In the morning, you will have 6 ounces of wonderful Yogurt Cream Cheese. The liquid that has drained into the bowl is whey, and can be used in soup or in baking as a substitute for buttermilk.

The Yogurt Cream Cheese can be spread on celery, on muffins or bagels, plain or mixed with fruit conserves, nuts, spices, or flavorings.

*Yield:* 6 ounces

---

**Each tablespoon provides approximately 20 calories.**

---

# Festive Figs

12 dried whole figs
⅓ cup chopped almonds
⅓ cup wheat sprouts (page 33)
½ cup dry sherry or apple juice
½ cup chopped sunflower seeds

Make a slit in one side of each fig. Mix almonds with wheat sprouts. Stuff each fig with the mixture.

Place stuffed figs in a bowl and cover with sherry or apple juice. Let stand for 24 hours, turning figs occasionally. Drain. Roll each fig lightly in chopped sunflower seeds.

*Yield:* 12 stuffed figs

---

**Each stuffed fig provides approximately 79 calories, 1.7 g protein, .3 g saturated fat, 3.7 g unsaturated fat, 1.2 mg sodium.**

---

## HOW TO GROW WHEAT SPROUTS

Put 4 tablespoons of wheat grains (available at health-food stores and some supermarkets) in a pint jar. Give them a quick rinse to remove surface dirt, then fill the jar two-thirds full with tepid water. Cover and let stand overnight. The next morning, cover the jar with two layers of cheesecloth secured with a rubber band, or with a screened lid available at gourmet and health-food stores. You can make your own from a window screen cut to fit a jar ring.

Without removing the screened lid, pour off the soak water, but do not discard it. Use it in soup or in cooking water for vegetables, or to replace the fat in a stir-fry.

Next, rinse the grains with tepid water, pour off the rinse water (give it to your plants), and let the jar rest under the sink or on the sink, slightly tilted so excess moisture can drain off. Use a sponge or folded dishcloth to prop up the jar bottom. Cover the jar with a tea towel if you're keeping it on the sink—the grains germinate best in the dark.

Repeat the rinsing procedure two or three times throughout the next two days. By the end of the second day, your wheat sprouts should be almost as long as the grain and ready for use. Refrigerate or freeze until you're ready to use them.

Follow the same procedure for other grains such as triticale and rye and for garbanzos (chick-peas).

# Peanut Butter and Carrot Sandwich

When was the last time you had a peanut butter sandwich? As any nut lover will attest, they're not just for kids. Protein-rich peanuts combined with carrots, the most popular member of the beta-carotene family, make for a super healthy duo. Use tahini (sesame butter) in place of the peanut butter if you like. The whole wheat bread also provides vitamin E as part of the important whole-grain family.

  ½ teaspoon linseed or olive oil
  1 tablespoon natural peanut butter
  4 slices whole-grain bread
  1 medium carrot, scrubbed and grated, raw or lightly cooked

Combine the oil with peanut butter and spread over one side of 2 slices of bread. Top with grated carrot. Close with the other 2 slices of bread. If you're in a rush to get to school or to work, pop the sandwich in a plastic bag and take it with you.

For a special treat on those mornings when you do have a few extra minutes, enjoy the sandwich grilled. After you assemble it, spread a smidgen of butter on the top side. Place the sandwich butter-side down on a hot skillet for about 3 minutes. Turn and grill the flip side for another 2 minutes.

*Yield:* 2 sandwiches

---

**Each sandwich provides approximately 300 calories, 8 g protein, 30 g unsaturated fat, 70 g sodium.**

---

*Variations:* Top peanut butter with bananas or apple or applesauce and sunflower seeds.

# Quick Party Pizzas

Great for impromptu parties. While your taste buds are celebrating, your body is welcoming its guardian angel, lycopene, provided by the tomato sauce, and your bad cholesterol is taking a nose dive, courtesy of your redolent friend, Mr. Garlic.

Whole wheat or rye bread or whole wheat pita
Garlic clove, peeled and halved
Tomato sauce or spaghetti sauce
Mozzarella or any good melting cheese
Oregano
Wheat sprouts (page 33)

Toast one slice of bread for each person. Rub each slice with half a garlic clove. Spread tomato or spaghetti sauce on each slice and cover with shredded cheese, oregano, and wheat sprouts. Place under the broiler or in a toaster oven until the cheese melts. For finger food, cut each slice into four portions. Serve immediately.

*Yield:* 4 little pizza fingers to each slice of whole wheat bread

---

**Each little pizza provides approximately 32 calories, 1.6 g protein, .5 g saturated fat, .3 g unsaturated fat, 30 mg sodium.**

---

# Spicy Bean Muffins

You won't believe how delicious a bean muffin can be! Not only are these muffins high in protein and fiber and low in calories, they lower your cholesterol in two ways. They contain beans, oat bran, and pectin, which lower cholesterol, and they're made with olive oil, which has been shown to lower LDL, the harmful cholesterol, without affecting HDL, the good cholesterol.

1 cup cooked, mashed pinto beans

1 egg

3 tablespoons olive or canola oil

1 teaspoon vanilla

2 tablespoons molasses or honey

½ cup sifted whole wheat pastry
   flour minus 2 tablespoons

2 tablespoons soy flour

2 tablespoons oat bran

2 tablespoons lecithin granules

½ teaspoon baking soda

½ teaspoon ground cinnamon

⅛ teaspoon ground nutmeg

⅛ teaspoon ground cloves

1 cup diced apples

½ cup raisins

¼ cup chopped nuts

In a mixing bowl or food processor, combine the beans, egg, oil, vanilla, and molasses or honey.

In another bowl, combine the flours, oat bran, lecithin, baking soda, and spices.

Preheat the oven to 350°F. Grease a regular-size tin for 12 muffins with nonstick cooking spray or line them with foil cups.

Add the dry ingredients to the bean mixture and mix briefly to combine ingredients. Stir in the apples, raisins, and nuts.

Spoon the batter into a muffin tin and bake for 20 minutes.

*Yield:* 12 muffins

Each muffin provides approximately 114 calories, 5 g protein, 1.6 g saturated fat, 11 g unsaturated fat, 19 mg sodium.

# Nut and Raisin Sprout Balls

When you sprout a seed or grain, its antioxidant values skyrocket.

   1 cup wheat or rye sprouts (page 33)
   1 cup pecans or other nuts or sunflower seeds
   1 cup raisins
   1 tablespoon honey
   Coconut crumbs, unsweetened, or ground almonds

In a food processor using the steel blade, grind sprouts, nuts or seeds, and raisins. Add honey and mix well. Form into 1-inch balls and roll in the coconut or ground almonds.

*Yield:* About 3 dozen

---

**Each sprout ball provides approximately 36 calories, 2 g protein, 2.9 g unsaturated fat, practically no sodium.**

---

# Sprouted Wheat Sticks

A delicious, crunchy bread stick. The sprouted wheat provides vitamin E, a powerhouse antioxidant that enhances the anticancer potential of selenium provided by the egg. The caraway seeds provide protease inhibitors that can help prevent or arrest cancer at the cellular level.

   3 cups sprouted wheat berries
   ¼ cup caraway seeds
   1 egg, lightly beaten
   Cornmeal

Grind the wheat berries in a meat grinder or food processor. Mix with the caraway seeds and the egg.

With moistened hands, work mixture into cigar shapes, roll in cornmeal, and place on a baking sheet spritzed with nonstick baking spray. Let dry for 5 minutes.

Preheat oven to 400°F.

Bake the wheat sticks for 10 minutes, then reduce heat to 325°F and continue baking about 5 minutes longer. These can be enjoyed hot, warm, or cold.

**Yield:** 12 sticks

---

**Each stick provides approximately 36 calories, 3 g protein, .5 g unsaturated fat, 20 mg sodium.**

---

# Baked Potato Pizza

There's nutritional gold in baked potatoes—potassium, magnesium, traces of the B vitamins, some calcium, and almost as much cancer-fighting vitamin C as you get in half a grapefruit. The pizza sauce provides jewels of cancer-fighting lycopene, more go-power, and lots of pizzazz. The combo also provides fiber and good complex carbohydrates that keep your body's motor running in high gear.

> 2 good-size baked potatoes
> ½ cup tomato or spaghetti sauce
> Oregano to taste
> 2 tablespoons grated part-skim mozzarella cheese

Cut the potatoes in halves, the long way. Top each with 2 tablespoons of tomato or spaghetti sauce, a big pinch of oregano, and a tablespoon of cheese. Broil in a toaster oven until cheese is melted. Enjoy.

## MICROWAVE METHOD

Assemble the potatoes as above and microcook on high, uncovered, for 2 minutes.

*Yield:* 2 to 4 servings

---

**Each half potato portion provides 93 calories, 4 g protein, 1.5 g saturated fat, 1 g unsaturated fat.**

---

# Baked Potato Skins

Rich in minerals, deliciously crunchy, high fiber, rich in antioxidants—all of this and mouthwatering too.

⅓ cup wheat germ
1 teaspoon chili powder
½ teaspoon ground cumin
½ teaspoon garlic powder

4 potatoes (about 8 ounces each),
    baked and cooled
¼ cup nonfat mayonnaise

Heat oven to 425°F. Spritz a cookie sheet with cooking spray.

Combine wheat germ, chili powder, cumin, and garlic powder on a piece of wax paper.

Cut potatoes in quarters lengthwise. Scoop out pulp, leaving ¼-inch thick shells. Brush shells very lightly with mayonnaise, then coat in the wheat germ mixture.

Bake on cookie sheet 25 minutes. Turn over, bake 25 minutes longer, or until crisp.

*Yield:* 4 servings

---

**Each serving provides approximately 84 calories, 3 g protein, 1 g fat, 309 mg sodium.**

---

# Sweet Potato Casserole

The hard-working lycopene in the tomatoes joins hands with the beta-carotene provided so generously by the sweet potatoes, making this dish a marriage of anticancer nutrients.

    2 tablespoons olive or canola oil
    4 cups raw, unpeeled sweet potato (about 3 potatoes), coarsely grated
    1 cup chopped onions
    ½ teaspoon cumin
    2 teaspoons paprika
    3 firm tomatoes, sliced ½ inch thick

In a large skillet, heat the oil over medium heat. Add sweet potato and onion, and sauté for about 4 minutes, until vegetables are crisp but tender. Add cumin and paprika and remove from heat.

Preheat oven to 350°F.

Spritz a shallow baking dish large enough to hold the tomatoes in a single layer with nonstick cooking spray. Place tomatoes in baking dish. Spoon the sweet potato mixture evenly over tomatoes.

Bake for about 15 minutes, until tomatoes are slightly softened.

*Yield:* 6 servings

---

**Each serving provides approximately 153 calories, 3 g protein, .6 g saturated fat, 4 g unsaturated fat, 12 mg sodium.**

---

## SWEET POTATOES

Did you ever realize as you dipped your fork into the deep orange flesh of a delicious sweet potato that not only were your taste buds dancing a jig, but also your body's defense system was cheering the arrival of 23,000 IU (14 mg) of beta-carotene that immediately went to work fortifying your defenses against macular degeneration, stroke, many kinds of cancers, and even heart disease?

Just take a gander at these headlines:

"CAROTENOIDS LINKED TO LOW RISK OF HEART DISEASE"
>—*Journal of the American Medical Association*, 9 November 1994

"BETA-CAROTENE = ANTIOXIDANT ARMOR, PROTECTS THE CELLS FROM THE KIND OF DAMAGE THAT CAN CAUSE CANCER"
>—*American Journal of Clinical Nutrition*, February 1994

"CAROTENOIDS LOWER THE INCIDENCE OF AGE-RELATED MAC-ULAR DEGENERATION"
>—Dr. Madison Dixon, optometrist, reported in *Miracle Cures* by Jean Carper

A half cup a day of sweet potatoes or its cousins in the squash and pumpkin family is health insurance with a delightful flavor.

# Shimmering Tuna in Aspic

A lovely dish that can be made ahead for very special occasions. The essential fatty acids in fish keep your heart on a steady track.

Two 6½-ounce cans albacore white tuna in water

3 tablespoons unflavored gelatin

Water

One 20-ounce can unsweetened crushed pineapple

3 tablespoons lemon juice

1 teaspoon grated lemon peel

1 tomato

1 cup plain yogurt

2 teaspoons vegetable seasoning

2 teaspoons prepared horseradish

1 teaspoon crumbled dill weed

¾ pound spinach, cooked and chopped

½ cup chopped green onions

Watercress or parsley for garnish

Drain tuna. Reserve the liquid. Sprinkle 1 tablespoon of gelatin over 1 cup cold water. Heat until gelatin dissolves. Cook until mixture reaches consistency of unbeaten egg white. Stir in 1 cup undrained pineapple, 1 tablespoon lemon juice, and the lemon peel. Pour into a 2-quart mold. Cut tomato in thin wedges. Stand wedges around the sides of the mold, anchoring them into the pineapple mixture. Refrigerate until set.

Drain the remaining pineapple, reserving juice. Add water to reserved juice to make 1¾ cups liquid. Sprinkle the remaining 2 tablespoons of gelatin over this liquid. Heat until gelatin dissolves. Remove from heat; cool slightly. Beat in yogurt, remaining 2 tablespoons lemon juice, vegetable seasonings, horseradish, and dill weed. Measure out 1 cup and set aside. Chill remaining mixture until it begins to thicken. Fold in tuna and pineapple. Pour over the set pineapple mixture. Refrigerate until set.

Pour reserved cup of yogurt mixture into food processor. Add cooked spinach and onions. Process until pureed. Pour over tuna mixture. Cover with plastic wrap. Chill until firm. Unmold on serving plate. Garnish with watercress or parsley.

*Yield:* 6 to 8 servings

Each serving provides approximately 99 calories, 18 g protein, a mere trace of fat, 44.5 mg sodium.

# Apricot-Mango Cole Slaw

Mango, the tropical fruit with the red and yellow jacket, is bursting with beta-carotene. In fact one medium mango provides more than 150 percent of the RDA. What's more, one mango harbors nearly 7 grams of fiber. Tossed with apricots, another beta-carotene superstar, and cabbage, a member of the cruciferous family, which claims more anti-cancer activists than any other vegetable, this is a superb sidedish.

3 cups shredded cabbage, red or
   green
1 carrot, pared and grated
3 tablespoons chopped onion
3 tablespoons chopped red, yellow,
   or green peppper
1 mango, peeled and diced
8 ounces apricot-mango nonfat
   yogurt

1 teaspoon caraway or celery
   seeds
2 tablespoons apple cider vinegar
½ teaspoon dry mustard
Freshly ground pepper to taste
½ teaspoon Salt-Free Herbal
   Seasoning (page 143)

In a large bowl, combine all ingredients and stir well.

*Yield:* 4 servings

Each serving provides approximately 110 calories, 4.5 g protein, .5 g fat, 55 mg sodium.

# Zippy Roasted Asparagus

2 tablespoons sesame or canola oil
½ teaspoon Dijon mustard
1 pound asparagus, washed and trimmed
Juice of ½ lemon

Preheat oven to 500°F.

In a small dish gradually whisk the oil into mustard. Place the asparagus in a roasting pan and toss it with the mustard mixture, until the spears are well coated. Roast until tender, shaking the pan several times. Depending on the size and age of the asparagus, timing will be about 8 to 11 minutes.

Transfer to a serving plate and squeeze lemon juice to taste over the asparagus.

*Yield:* 4 servings

---

**Each serving provides approximately 91.5 calories, 3.6 g protein, 1 g saturated fat, 6 g unsaturated fat, 6 mg sodium.**

---

# Avocado with Cauliflower and Almonds

A good health anticancer trio: avocado, cauliflower, and almonds. Avocadoes contribute a bonanza of vitamins, minerals, and essential fatty acids to this dish. One-half of an avocado contains only 150 calories and provides 290 units of vitamin A, an important antioxidant that quenches free radicals that cause premature aging, cancer, and cardiovascular disease. Cauliflower is a member of the cruciferous vegetable family, which provides protection against many cancers, notably cancer of the colon, stomach, prostate, and bladder. Almonds contribute protein, several B vitamins, calcium, iron, potassium, and a delicious crunch.

1 avocado, peeled and pitted
1 tablespoon grated onion
1 tablespoon lemon juice
1 tablespoon minced parsley
1 head cauliflower, cut into florets
3 tablespoons slivered almonds

In a medium bowl, mash the avocado, and add the onion, lemon juice, and minced parsley. Steam the cauliflower until fork-tender. Spoon avocado mixture over the hot cauliflower and top with slivered almonds. Serve immediately.

*Yield:* 6 servings

Each serving provides approximately 85 calories, 2 g protein, 1.35 g saturated fat, 8 g unsaturated fat, 7.5 mg sodium.

# Green Beans Almondine

I find that children and other vegetable scorners go for seconds of green beans when they're topped with tempting toasted nuts.

  2 teaspoons dried dill
  4 teaspoons lemon juice
  1 teaspoon unsalted butter
  1 pound green beans, steamed
  1 tablespoon slivered almonds, lightly toasted

In a small nonstick skilled, combine dill, lemon juice, and butter. Heat until butter melts. Place the steamed beans in a serving bowl and drizzle with the dill mixture. Sprinkle the toasted almonds on top.

*Yield:* 8 servings

---

**Each serving provides 26 calories, .6 g fat, 11 mg sodium.**

---

# Broccoli and Onions with Yogurt-Cheese Sauce

The combination of flavors and textures in this anticancer bonanza make getting healthy a real pleasure even George Bush would enjoy.

The broccoli, onion, and yogurt deliver their significant protective potential. Keep this healthy thought in mind as you enjoy this dish.

One 10-ounce package frozen cut
  broccoli, or 2 cups lightly cooked
  chopped fresh broccoli
1 medium onion, peeled and cut
  into 16 wedges
1 tablespoon water

½ cup Yogurt Cream Cheese (page 32)
1 teaspoon arrowroot powder
¼ teaspoon lemon juice
¼ teaspoon crushed dried basil
⅛ teaspoon dried rosemary,
  crushed

In a 1½-quart casserole, combine broccoli, onion, and water. Microcook on high, covered, for 5 to 6 minutes, or until broccoli is crisp-tender. Drain.

In a small bowl, combine the yogurt cheese, arrowroot, lemon juice, basil, and rosemary. Mix well. Microcook, uncovered, on high for 2 to 3 minutes, or till thickened and bubbly. Pour cheese mixture over broccoli.

*Yield:* 4 servings

Each serving provides approximately 48 calories, 5 g protein, .5 g saturated fat, .4 g unsaturated fat, 35 mg sodium.

# Marinated Beets in Creamy Yogurt

Beets contain antioxidant vitamins A and C, also energizing B vitamins and fair amounts of calcium, iron, magnesium, and phosphorous. Raspberries are a deliciously flavorful source of fiber, vitamin C, and heart-savvy potassium.

One 15-ounce can of beets, or 2 cups cooked fresh beets, cut into julienne
½ cup Raspberry Vinaigrette (page 142)
1 cup nonfat plain yogurt

Marinate the beets in the vinaigrette for several hours, turning frequently. About an hour before serving, drain the beets (save the marinade and use as salad dressing) and toss with the yogurt.

*Yield:* 4 servings

Each serving provides approximately 56 calories, 2.5 g protein, 1.5 g saturated fat, 2 g unsaturated fat, 46 mg sodium.

## EXPAND YOUR VEGETABLE HORIZONS

How many different vegetables have you enjoyed in the past month? Bet you could count them on the fingers of one hand and have two fingers left over.

If this has been your custom, then let me help you branch out and discover the great big wonderful world of vegetables. You will not only experience some new gustatory pleasures, but you will also reap many health dividends that researchers are only now finding deep in the heart of the vegetable kingdom.

Vegetables are a good source of beta-carotene, which has been shown to inhibit the development of cancerous growths. And that's not all. Many are rich in soluble fiber, the kind that has been shown to lower cholesterol levels and contribute to the health of the cardiovascular system. They're also rich in insoluble fiber, which is linked to healthy colons. They are rich in vitamins, minerals, and very low in calories.

How can you best prepare vegetables to conserve their color, texture, flavor, and nutrient values?

Since light and air can destroy vitamins, it is best to store your vegetables in a dark place where there is little moisture loss. The ideal place is the humidifier drawer of your refrigerator. Also, the larger the exposed surface, the greater the loss of vitamins. Therefore, chop or slice vegetables when you are ready to eat or cook them, not a day or an hour ahead of time.

Water-soluble vitamins C and B leach out into the cooking water. Heat too is destructive. Therefore, cook vegetables as briefly as possible and in as little water as possible.

Since there will be some unavoidable losses caused by cooking, always serve some vegetables raw, even though you may be serving the same vegetables cooked. Prepare a beautiful salad of leafy greens. Use romaine, spinach, cabbage, radishes, scallions, mushrooms, sliced zucchini, and whatever else is available. You'll be surprised how people gobble up the same vegetables in the raw that are scorned when they are cooked.

Remember that the liquid in which vegetables are cooked contains some water-soluble vitamins and minerals and should never be discarded. Use it in soups or drink it.

---

# Broccoflower with Brazil Nuts

The offspring of a broccoli mother and cauliflower father, broccoflower provides more of some antioxidants than its parents.

In flavor and appearance, broccoflower is reminiscent of both its parents, less cabbagelike than cauliflower, crisply green like broccoli. It has as much vitamin C as broccoli, three times more than cauliflower, and twice as much beta-carotene as cauliflower. Use broccoflower as you would either of its parents. Steam it, with bay leaf, basil, thyme, or rosemary added to the cooking water or stock.

Brazil nuts are an excellent source of selenium.

1 tablespoon olive or canola oil

2 tablespoons chopped Brazil nuts

1 pound broccoflower trimmed, peeled, and cut into florets, lightly steamed
(or substitute a combination of broccoli and cauliflower, or use either one
separately)

1 teaspoon reduced sodium soy sauce

1 teaspoon rice wine or Balsamic vinegar

In a large frying pan, heat the oil, add the Brazil nuts to toast briefly. Add the broccoflower and mix with the nuts. Toss with the soy sauce and rice wine.

*Yield:* 4 servings

---

**Each serving provides 54 calories, 4 g protein .6 g unsaturated fat, 17 mg sodium.**

---

# Broccoli Pudding

I love it when my family asks for seconds of this dish because whether or not they realize it, they're getting second helpings of beta-carotene, vitamin C, selenium, potassium, and folic acid, all of which help them to enjoy better health and stay looking young longer.

1½ cups cooked broccoli, drained

1 tablespoon butter, melted

½ teaspoon, crushed dried oregano

⅛ teaspoon freshly ground pepper

1 teaspoon Salt-Free Herbal
Seasoning (page 143)

⅓ cup oat bran or wheat germ or a
combination

4 eggs

2 cups milk

Lightly butter or coat with nonstick cooking spray a 1-quart baking dish.

Preheat the oven to 325°F. Place a pan of water large enough to hold the 1-quart dish in the oven. Allow it to heat while preparing the pudding.

In a food processor, using the metal blade, finely chop the broccoli. Add the butter, seasonings, and oat bran or wheat germ. Blend to combine ingredients. Add the eggs and run the machine for 8 seconds, scraping down the sides as needed. With the machine running, pour 1 cup of milk through the feed tube and continue blending 3 more seconds.

Pour the broccoli mixture into the prepared baking dish. Return the bowl and blade to the food processor base and add the remaining milk. Turn the machine on and off twice. (This will mix the milk with the particles of the batter that cling to the bowl and blade. It also contributes to the formation of the tasty pudding layer.) Pour over the mixture in the baking dish and stir gently until well mixed.

Carefully place the baking dish in the preheated water bath and bake for 60 minutes, or until a knife inserted into the center comes out clean.

*Yield:* 6 servings

---

**Each serving provides approximately 158 calories, 11.5 g protein, 3.5 g saturated fat, 4 g unsaturated fat, 98 mg sodium.**

---

# Brussels Sprouts with Grapes

These miniature cabbages are a member of the cruciferous vegetable family, a group that is highly valued for their indole content which has been shown to block the action of cancer agents. Grapes, like most fruits, contain phenols which have considerable anti-cancer power.

1 pint fresh Brussels sprouts

1 tablespoon unsalted butter

¼ cup chopped onion

¼ cup finely chopped celery

2 tablespoons soy flour

1¾ cups low-fat milk

2 tablespoons lemon juice

1 teaspoon Salt-Free Herbal
  Seasoning (page 143)

¼ teaspoon dried leaf marjoram

2 cups seedless green grapes

Steam the Brussels sprouts for about 8 minutes, or until crisp-tender.

In a large saucepan, melt the butter. Add onion and celery and cook until tender. Sprinkle the flour over the onion and celery and toss to combine. Gradually stir in the milk and continue to stir until mixture comes to a boil and thickens.

Stir in the lemon juice, seasoning, marjoram, grapes, and the cooked Brussels sprouts. Cook until thoroughly heated.

*Yield:* 8 servings

---

**Each serving provides approximately 81 calories, 4.4 g protein, 7.4 g saturated fat, trace of unsaturated fat, 36 mg sodium.**

---

# Fruit and Cabbage Salad with Honey-Caraway Dressing

The wonderful hard-working indoles in the cabbage provide compounds that deactivate potent estrogens that stimulate the growth of some tumors; flavonoids in the orange protect your cells from free radical damage; abundant beta-carotene in the apricots offers cancer protection and may prevent plaque deposits in your arteries. Just think of this powerful triumvirate working for you as you enjoy every bite.

4 cups finely shredded green or purple cabbage

1 cup orange sections

½ cup diced dried apricots

Parsley sprigs for garnish

Honey-Caraway Dressing (page 138)

Chill all ingredients. At serving time combine all ingredients except parsley and pile into a salad bowl. Garnish with parsley sprigs. Serve with Honey-Caraway Dressing.

*Yield:* 6 servings

---

**Each serving provides approximately 56 calories, 1.3 g protein, no fat, 3.3 mg sodium.**

---

# Caraway Cabbage

Cabbage is far more versatile than we are led to believe: Most often used for cole slaw, I especially like it on its own, slightly cooked and herbed judiciously. Not only is it a good source of vitamins C and A—both protective antioxidants—calcium, and potassium, but it is a boon to waist watchers with only 20 calories in a whole cup.

The cayenne provides capsaicin, an anti-inflammatory that has been used to treat cluster headaches (Earl Mindell's *Food as Medicine*).

2 tablespoons unsalted butter or oil

2 cups finely sliced cabbage
   (1 small head)

¼ cup water

1 cup low-fat sour cream or yogurt

1 tablespoon slightly crushed
   caraway seeds

½ teaspoon kelp

Cayenne pepper to taste

Heat 2 tablespoons butter or oil in a wide frying pan on high heat. Add the cabbage and the water. Cover and cook, stirring occasionally for 3 to 4 minutes. Season to taste. You could serve it this way or fancy it up by draining off the liquid, then adding sour cream or yogurt, caraway seeds, kelp, and cayenne.

*Yield:* 4 servings

---

Each serving provides approximately 91 calories, 2.5 g protein, 3.5 g saturated fat, 2.1 g unsaturated fat, 41 mg sodium.

---

# Carrot Kugel

Even those who scorn vegetables reach for a second helping of this delicious kugel. Serve it hot or cold, with chicken and a salad for a meal rich in life-saving antioxidants.

2 large carrots, pared and grated
2 tablespoons canola, olive, or
    peanut oil
2 eggs, separated
¼ cup honey
¼ cup soy flour
¾ cup whole wheat pastry flour

½ teaspoon baking powder
1 teaspoon vanilla extract
3 teaspoons grated lemon rind
½ cup raisins
½ cup sunflower seeds or chopped
    walnuts

Preheat the oven to 350°F. Coat a loaf pan with nonstick cooking spray. In a bowl, combine the carrots, oil, egg yolks, and honey. Add the flours, baking powder, vanilla, grated rind, raisins, and seeds or nuts. Beat the egg whites until stiff and fold into the flour mixture. Bake for 35 minutes or until golden brown.

*Yield:* 6 servings

---

Each serving provides approximately 254 calories, 4.5 g protein, 1.2 g saturated fat, 6 g unsaturated fat, 31 mg sodium.

---

# Carrots and Yogurt

A lovely marriage of colors and anticancer forces.

1 large carrot, pared and cut into
   1½-inch julienne
1 cup yogurt
1 teaspoon honey
¼ teaspoon ground cumin

¼ cup finely chopped onion
½ teaspoon crushed hot red pepper
   flakes, or ¼ teaspoon cayenne
   pepper.

Cut the carrot pieces lengthwise into very thin slices. Stack the slices and cook for about a half minute. Drain well.

Combine the yogurt, carrot, and remaining ingredients. Serve chilled as a side dish.

*Yield:* About 1¹/₂ cups

---

Each ¹/₄-cup portion provides approximately 33 calories, 1.7 g protein, just a trace of fat, 16 mg sodium.

---

# Crunchy Carrot Balls

A delicious wholesome snack, rich in beta-carotene and other cancer inhibitors from the yogurt cream cheese, orange zest, and parsley.

½ cup Yogurt Cream Cheese (page 32)
1 teaspoon honey
1 cup shredded carrots
⅓ cup Grape-Nuts cereal
1 tablespoon orange zest
2 tablespoons finely chopped parsley

In medium-size bowl or in bowl of food processor, combine cheese and honey until well blended. Stir in the shredded carrots.

Cover and chill for 30 minutes. Form into one-inch balls. Cover and chill.

On a piece of wax paper, combine the Grape-Nuts cereal, orange zest, and parsley. Just before serving, roll balls in the cereal mixture.

*Yield:* 15 one-inch balls

---

**Each ball provides approximately 15 calories, .7 g protein, 13 mg (a mere trace) of fat, 13 mg sodium.**

---

# Cauliflower Kugel

This sensational pudding will lend pizzazz to a fish or fowl dinner or, topped with melting cheese, is a great vegetarian meal that provides cancer-deterrent indoles, beta-carotenes, selenium, and some vitamin E.

1 large head of cauliflower, trimmed
and separated into florets

1 medium-size onion, diced

2 eggs

¼ teaspoon white pepper

¼ teaspoon nutmeg

⅓ cup wheat germ, whole wheat
flour, or oat bran

3 tablespoons olive or canola oil

Sesame seeds for garnish

Preheat oven to 350°F.

In a food processor, using metal blade, combine cauliflower, onion, eggs, pepper, and nutmeg. Process until cauliflower is finely chopped. Add the wheat germ, flour, or oat bran and the oil and process briefly. Turn the mixture into a well-greased 9-inch square baking dish. Top with sesame seeds. Bake for about 1 hour, until golden brown and crisp. Serve with applesauce or yogurt.

*Yield:* 6 servings

---

**Each serving provides approximately 121 calories, 6.3 g protein, 1.4 g saturated fat, 7 g unsaturated fat, 26 mg sodium.**

---

# Chestnut and Cranberry Stuffing

Enjoy a rainbow of life-enhancing phytochemicals in every delicious bite.

1 quart cranberries

2 tablespoons olive or canola oil

½ cup minced onion

1 cup sliced celery

4 cloves garlic, minced

¼ cup sliced mushrooms

2 tablespoons honey

3 cups cooked brown rice

2 cups chestnuts, canned or fresh,
cooked, and peeled

1 teaspoon ground coriander

1 teaspoon dried sage

1 teaspoon dried, crushed rosemary

2 teaspoons dried oregano

Soak cranberries in very hot water for 5 minutes, then drain and set aside.

In a large skillet, heat the oil, and sauté the onion, celery, garlic, and mushrooms over medium heat, just until vegetables are limp.

In a large bowl, combine the sautéed vegetables, cranberries, honey, rice, chestnuts, coriander, sage, rosemary, and oregano.

Transfer the stuffing ingredients to a 3-quart baking dish spritzed with nonstick cooking spray. Cover and bake at 350°F for about 30 minutes.

*Yield:* 10 servings

---

**Each serving provides approximately 205 calories, 2.5 g protein, 3.4 g fat, 14 mg sodium.**

---

# Chilled Eggplant with Tomatoes

At potluck parties, this dish attracts the biggest circle of enthusiastic nibblers. I wonder if they know how healthy they are getting. Tomatoes provide lycopene, a very effective antioxidant. Cooking actually increases the effectiveness of lycopene.

> 1 eggplant
> 3 tomatoes, chopped
> 3 tablespoons olive oil
> 1 tablespoon vinegar
> 1 tablespoon honey
> Pepper to taste

Preheat the oven to 350°F. Place the eggplant on a baking sheet and bake for 25 to 30 minutes. Let cool and peel the eggplant. Chop into small cubes. In a medium bowl combine the eggplant and the remaining ingredients. Chill for 1 hour. Serve with crackers or toasted whole wheat pita bread cut in triangles.

*Yield:* 6 servings

Each serving provides approximately 70 calories, 1.3 g protein, .4 g saturated fat, 4 g unsaturated fat, 6 mg sodium.

# Baked Garlic Potatoes

Irresistibly good. The garlic, the parsley, and the oil do many good things for the body. The fragrance of this dish nourishes the soul.

1 pound small potatoes
5 cloves garlic, minced
4 tablespoons olive oil
¼ cup chopped parsley
2 teaspoons Salt-Free Herbal Seasoning (page 143)
¼ teaspoon freshly ground pepper

Preheat oven to 450°F. Wash and dry potatoes. Arrange in a casserole in two layers. Combine garlic, oil, parsley, herbal seasoning, and pepper. Pour over potatoes and toss to coat with oil mixture.

Bake for 20 minutes. Turn potatoes to recoat with the oil mixture, then bake another 20 minutes. Cut potatoes open and squeeze the ends to fluff them up.

*Yield:* 6 servings

Each serving provides approximately 120 calories, 1.5 g protein, 1.5 g saturated fat, 9 mg sodium.

## GARLIC: THE PUNGENT HEALTH PROTECTOR

Garlic, part of the lily family along with onions, leeks, and chives, may be biting to the taste buds and impudent to the nostrils, but when it comes to performing countless pharmaceutical functions, and blocking some of the most vicious cancer-causing agents, garlic may exude the sweet smell of succor.

It has long been known that garlic tends to lower high blood pressure levels slightly. It affects high serum cholesterol by reducing only the harmful LDL and leaving the protective HDL at normal levels; it reduces levels of triglycerides, and slows blood coagulation time, thus reducing clotting.

And now, research reveals that garlic may lessen the incidence of cancers of the stomach, liver, lungs, breast, esophagus, colon, and rectum.

Here are some suggestions to help you get more of this therapeutic wonder food in your diet:

- Rub a cut clove over your salad bowl every time you use it.
- Crushed garlic sautéed in a little olive oil makes a tasty topping for cooked broccoli or cauliflower.
- Mince a clove of garlic into a cup of plain yogurt. Add a teaspoon each of chopped dill, parsley, and scallions for a tangy dip or salad dressing.
- Rub a cut clove of garlic on marrow and meat bones headed for the soup pot—and skip the salt.
- Mince a clove of garlic into your ground meat when you're making patties, meat loaf, or meatballs.

Delicious!

# Scrumptious Garlic Mashed Potatoes

It just so happens that this great American comfort food is a storehouse of anticancer fighters. Indulge.

4 medium potatoes (about 1½ pounds)

1 cup milk

1 tablespoon unsalted butter

3 cloves garlic, minced

Kelp or Salt-Free Herbal Seasoning (page 143) to taste

Freshly ground pepper to taste

Chopped parsley, for garnish

After scrubbing and patting the potatoes dry, pierce each one all over with a fork.

Bake them in an oven at 400°F for about an hour or microcook them on high for about 13 minutes. Halve lengthwise; scoop out pulp into a medium-size microsafe bowl.

Mash potatoes or beat with an electric mixer.

In a measuring cup or microsafe bowl, combine milk, butter, and garlic. Microwave on high for 2 minutes. Mix into potato pulp. Season to taste with kelp or herbal seasoning and pepper.

Microcook on high for 1 minute. Sprinkle with chopped parsley, serve at once, and watch those faces light up.

*Yield:* 4 servings

Each serving provides approximately 144 calories, 2.5 g protein, 3.3 g saturated fat, 2 g unsaturated fat, 3.1 mg sodium.

# Lemony Steamed Vegetables

Steam these in as little water as possible and take care not to overcook. The vegetables should be intensely bright.

6 small red-skin new potatoes, scrubbed and halved

¾ pound carrots, pared and sliced diagonally into ¼-inch pieces

¾ pound Brussels sprouts, trimmed

6 large cloves fresh garlic, peeled and sliced

1 teaspoon Salt-Free Herbal Seasoning (page 143)

2 bay leaves

3 lemon slices

2 tablespoons softened unsalted butter

1 teaspoon chopped parsley

1 chicken bouillon cube, crumbled

¼ teaspoon fresh savory, minced

¼ teaspoon fresh rosemary, minced

¼ teaspoon freshly ground pepper

Place vegetables in steamer basket in layers, sprinkling herbal seasonings and interspersing garlic cloves between layers. Top with bay leaves and lemon slices.

Steam for 20 to 30 minutes, or until vegetables are crisp-tender.

Meanwhile, blend together the butter, parsley, crumbled bouillon cube, savory, rosemary, and pepper.

Place the steamed vegetables in a bowl. Remove the garlic cloves and mash with the seasoned butter. Dot over vegetables and toss lightly to combine. Serve with remaining garlic cloves.

*Yield:* 4 servings

---

**Each serving provides approximately 158 calories, 3.6 g protein, 3 g saturated fat, 2 g unsaturated fat, 33 mg sodium.**

---

# Orange Bulgur with Pistachios

Bulgur is made from whole wheat berries that have been steamed, then dried and crushed. It is quick cooking and has a pleasant flavor, which in this recipe is enhanced by the orange juice. The juice provides vitamin C, and the pistachio nuts have protease inhibitors that may block the inception and progression of cancer.

2 cups orange juice
1 cup bulgur
¼ cup chopped pistachios or almonds

In a saucepan, bring the orange juice to a boil.

Add the bulgur and cook over lowered heat for 10 to 15 minutes. Add the nuts or pass them at the table.

*Yield:* 3 servings

Each serving with pistachios provides approximately 270 calories, 7 g protein, 3 g unsaturated fat, just a trace of sodium.

# Super Barley Pilaf

Apricots, nuts, and raisins combine with barley to make a sensational antioxidant- and phytochemical-rich pilaf that can double as a stuffing for poultry or fish while it enhances your protection from both cancer and heart disease.

| | |
|---|---|
| 2 tablespoons olive or canola oil | ½ cup chopped dried apricots |
| 1 medium onion, finely chopped | ⅓ cup chopped almonds, pine nuts, |
| 1 cup sliced fresh mushrooms |    or sunflower seeds |
| 1 cup raw barley | ⅓ cup raisins |
| 4 cups boiling water, or vegetable or | ¼ teaspoon white pepper |
|    chicken stock | 1 teaspoon cinnamon |

In a large heavy skillet, heat the oil and sauté onion and mushrooms slowly until mushrooms are soft and onion transparent. Remove to a covered dish.

In the same pan, sauté the barley briefly. Do not allow it to brown or burn. Three minutes should do it.

Add the boiling water or stock to the barley, then add the mushroom and onion mixture and the remaining ingredients. Do not stir. Cover the pot and simmer at low heat until all water is absorbed, about 1 hour. Stir mixture carefully, place a tea towel over the pot (to absorb excess moisture), and replace the lid. Allow to stand for 15 minutes before serving.

*Yield:* 4 to 6 servings as a pilaf; 4 cups of stuffing

---

**Each of 6 portions provides approximately 266 calories, 4 g protein, 1 g saturated fat, 7 g unsaturated fat, 10.4 mg sodium.**

---

# SOUPS AND STEWS

Creamy Apricot-Carrot Soup, redolent of flavors that are like a mother's embrace; Cabbage, Tomato, and Apple Soup, bursting with lusty flavors and invaluable antioxidants; Quick Vegetable Soup, made with six different vegetables, soy granules, and a lot of garlic . . . it makes you hungry, doesn't it?

When you have soup in the freezer or the refrigerator, you've got a hearty, handy, satisfying meal ready to reheat while you set the table.

Make your soup in a large pot. Place the portion that is not consumed in single portion containers and store in the freezer. When you come home tired and hungry, you've got it made.

## HEART-HEALTHY SOUPS

No matter what your mood, or your nutritional needs, soup can fill the bill. There's no better vehicle for enriching your body with important nutrients, for lifting your spirits, and for providing many of the nutrients that help prevent disease.

Soups can be hot, filling, cheering, satisfying, and custom made. They can provide trace minerals, vitamins, and fiber, all important to a healthy heart; and they can make you feel full and satisfied on very few calories.

There's much more to soup than a tantalizing aroma and a great blend of subtle flavors. Soup is the ideal replacement fluid. Because vegetables, grains, and meats release their goodness into the fluid in which they are steeped, soup contains everything one finds in plant and animal tissue.

The nutritive value of soup can be further increased by adding soy or peanut flour. These products are almost pure protein and yet are rich in vitamins, minerals, and antioxidants. Soup can contribute to your cholesterol-lowering program by the addition of oatmeal or oat bran. These products thicken the soup slightly but do not change the taste if used with a gentle hand. Flavor your soups with herbs like dill, parsley, bay leaves, vegetable seasoners, a bit of lemon juice, and go very easy on the salt or better yet, omit the salt and season with a sprinkle of cayenne, which provides the phytochemical capsaicin.

These soups will enhance the enjoyment of lunch or dinner and are seasoned with just enough bite to intrigue the tongue and please the palate and yet with nary a grain of salt.

# High-Mineral Broth

This broth provides a rainbow of valuable antioxidants and is a favorite at many health spas. If you prefer a clear broth, strain the liquid. I like to puree the whole thing in the food processor. This makes a thicker, but very hearty broth and will provide fiber as well as a gold mine of nutrients.

1 cup shredded carrots
1 tablespoon chopped parsley
1 tablespoon chopped chives
1 quart water
1 cup tomato juice, or 1 cup
   chopped tomatoes

1 teaspoon vegetable seasoning
1 teaspoon honey
1 tablespoon nutritional yeast
   (optional)

In a large soup pot, combine the shredded carrots, parsley, and chives with water. Cover and cook over medium heat for 30 minutes. Add tomato juice or tomatoes, vegetable seasoning, yeast if you're using it, and honey. Cook 5 minutes more.

### MICROWAVE METHOD

In a 2½-quart soufflé dish, combine the carrots, parsley, and chives and water. Cover and microcook on full power for 5 minutes. Add the tomato juice, vegetable seasoning, yeast if you're using it, and honey, and microcook, covered, for 1 minute and 30 seconds. Strain or puree in food processor.

*Yield:* 4 servings

---

**Each serving provides 30 calories, 2 g protein, no significant fat or sodium.**

---

# Garlic Soup

Credited with the ability to cure everything from toothaches to evil demons, garlic has recently been shown to lower blood glucose and cholesterol levels in addition to possessing cancer-fighting properties. Whenever you're under the weather, try a little of this heaven in a bowl.

| | |
|---|---|
| 6 cloves garlic, peeled | 1 bay leaf |
| Sprig of fresh sage, or ¼ teaspoon dried | 4 cups chicken or vegetable broth |
| Sprig of fresh thyme, or ¼ teaspoon dried | 1 cup Garlic Croutons (page 143) |
| | 1 beaten egg yolk |

Simmer garlic, sage, thyme, and bay leaf in broth for about 30 minutes. Remove from heat and strain, reserving garlic cloves. Add ½ cup croutons to broth and allow to sit about 10 minutes. Beat smooth. Smash reserved garlic cloves and add to thickened broth. Carefully add beaten egg yolk and reheat, but don't boil. Serve with remaining croutons sprinkled on top.

*Yield:* 6 servings

---

**Each serving provides insignificant calories.**

---

# Gazpacho

This refreshing chilled soup is super delicious and a veritable storehouse of antioxidant- and phytochemical-rich foods.

| | |
|---|---|
| 2 stalks celery | 2 tablespoons minced parsley |
| 2 carrots | 1 clove garlic, chopped |
| 4 green onions with tops | ½ teaspoon freshly ground pepper |
| 1 cucumber, pared | 3 tablespoons olive oil |
| 1 green or red pepper, halved and cored | 1 cup vegetable broth or water |
| | ¼ cup red wine vinegar |
| 4 medium-size tomatoes, halved and cored | 2 cups tomato or V-8 juice |
| | Plain yogurt |

Coarsely chop all of the vegetables in the food processor. Add the remaining ingredients and puree until smooth. Chill for a few hours or overnight. You may have to do this in two batches. Serve with a dollop of plain yogurt.

*Yield:* 7 servings

---

Each serving provides approximately 109 calories, 1.1 g protein, 1.4 g saturated fat, 5 g unsaturated fat, 132 mg sodium.

---

# Alfalfa Sprout Gazpacho

This version of gazpacho calls for a healthy dose of alfalfa sprouts. Alfalfa, whose name means "best food," sends its roots very deep into the ground where they pick up many valuable trace minerals—ten times the mineral value of most grains, says Dr. Bernard Jensen, D.C., author of *Seeds and Sprouts for Life.*

> 1 cup alfalfa sprouts
> 4 cups tomato juice
> ½ cucumber, chopped
> 1 green onion, chopped
> ½ green pepper, chopped
> 2 medium-size tomatoes, chopped

Combine all ingredients in blender or food processor and puree until smooth. Chill for an hour. Serve as a beverage or a soup.

*Yield:* 6 cups

---

Each cup provides approximately 51 calories, 3 g protein, no fat, 62 mg sodium.

---

# Quick Vegetable Soup

This hearty, flavorful soup is a good form of health insurance. Almost a dozen vegetables contribute to a cornucopia of antioxidants, each one doing a specific job that contributes to wiping out cancer-causing free radicals.

3 cups water or vegetable broth
½ teaspoon freshly ground pepper
1 teaspoon salt-free vegetable
   seasoner
2 cup grated vegetables (carrots,
   onions, zucchini, celery, turnips,
   rutabagas, etc.)

2 cups coarsely chopped greens
   (parsley, spinach, romaine, etc.)
2 tablespoons oat bran
2 tablespoons soy granules
3 cloves garlic, finely chopped
½ cup parsley, finely chopped
2 tablespoons unsalted butter

In a large soup pot, bring the water or vegetable broth, pepper, and vegetable seasoner to a boil.

Add the vegetables and cook for 5 minutes. Add the oat bran and soy granules, chopped garlic, parsley, and butter and bring to a boil. Season to taste and serve immediately.

If the soup is too thick, thin it with a little milk or yogurt.

*Yield:* 6 servings

---

**Each serving provides 125 calories, 2 g protein, 2 g saturated fat, 1.4 g unsaturated fat, 13 mg sodium.**

---

# Tomato Soup Topped with Avocado

The powerful lycopene in the tomatoes accompanied by the special antioxidant tributes of the avocado give you a double barrel of protection from the ravages of free radicals that cause aging, cancer, and cardiovascular disease, and all while you are happily enjoying a delicious bowl of soup.

10 plum tomatoes, diced

2 cups chicken or vegetable broth

2 cups chopped onions, preferably red

3 tablespoons tomato paste

3 cloves garlic, chopped or grated

1 teaspoon kelp

½ cup buttermilk or yogurt

2 tablespoons chopped parsley

½ teaspoon cayenne pepper or red pepper sauce

## Topping

1 cup diced avocado

1 cup diced cucumber

2 tablespoons diced red onion

Combine in a large soup pot the tomatoes, broth, onions, tomato paste, garlic, and kelp. Cover and simmer for about 45 minutes.

Puree in food processor. Transfer to a large bowl and stir in the buttermilk or yogurt, parsley, and cayenne or red pepper sauce.

To make the topping, combine the ingredients in a small bowl. Ladle the soup into serving bowls. Spoon some of the topping over each serving bowl.

This soup can be enjoyed either hot or cold.

*Yield:* 4 hearty servings

**Each serving provides 130 calories, 5 g protein, 22 g carbohydrates, 5 g unsaturated fat, 5 g fiber, negligible cholesterol, 500 mg sodium..**

# Cabbage, Tomato, and Apple Soup

This hearty soup is bursting with palate-pleasing lusty flavors and invaluable nutrients. Cabbage, a member of the cruciferous family, provides indoles, which help to nullify cancer-causing agents.

2 tablespoons olive oil

1 medium onion, chopped

1 clove garlic, minced

5 cups vegetable broth or water

3 cups shredded cabbage

1 potato, diced

2 apples, unpeeled, chopped

2 tomatoes, chopped

¼ teaspoon freshly ground pepper

In a large soup pot, heat the oil over medium heat. Sauté the onion and garlic for about a minute. Add all remaining ingredients and cook for about 25 minutes.

*Yield:* 7 servings

---

**Each serving provides 96 calories, 2.1 g protein, .5 g saturated fat, 3.5 g unsaturated fat, 2 mg sodium.**

---

# Vegetable Soup with Walnut Dumplings

Walnut dumplings, seasoned with garlic, parsley, sage, and marjoram and fortified with the yolk of an egg, give this hearty vegetable soup an extra culinary dimension fortified with antioxidants and protease inhibitors that offer cancer protection on several levels.

## Soup

2 quarts water or vegetable
   stock

1 carrot, pared and chopped

1 parsnip, or parsley root, pared
   and chopped

3 small potatoes, scrubbed and cut
   in quarters

2 stalks celery with tops, cut in
   1-inch pieces

1 clove garlic, minced

2 onions, quartered

1 teaspoon Salt-Free Herbal
   Seasoning (page 143)

Freshly ground pepper to taste

## Dumplings

1 tablespoon canola or olive oil, or
   butter

2 tablespoons finely minced onion

2 tablespoons whole wheat, rye, or
   spelt flour

2 tablespoons soy flour

4 tablespoons wheat germ

1 egg yolk

½ cup cold water

Pinch of garlic powder

Pinch of freshly ground pepper

1 slice whole-grain bread, soaked in
   water, then pressed out and torn
   into small pieces

2 tablespoons finely chopped
   walnuts

1 tablespoon finely chopped parsley

Pinch of marjoram or sage

1 egg white, beaten to soft peaks

3 cups water

### TO MAKE THE SOUP

In a large soup pot, heat the water or stock. Add the next 8 ingredients. Cover, bring to a boil, and simmer for 1 hour.

### TO MAKE THE DUMPLINGS

In a medium-size skillet, heat the oil or butter, add the minced onion, sauté until golden. Sprinkle the flours and wheat germ over the onion and sauté briefly.

In a bowl, beat the egg yolk with the cold water; add the garlic powder and pepper. Add this mixture to the onion mixture. Add the soaked bread, chopped nuts, parsley, and marjoram or sage. Let stand 15 minutes, then fold in the beaten egg white.

In a saucepan, bring the 3 cups of water to a boil. With a spoon take 1 tablespoon of the dumpling mixture and ease it into the boiling water. Repeat until the mixture is used up. Reduce the heat and simmer for 15 minutes, until the dumplings are light and fluffy. Remove the dumplings with a slotted spoon. Place a few in each soup bowl, and spoon the vegetables and soup over them.

*Yield:* 8 servings

---

Each serving of soup provides approximately 46 calories, 1.2 g protein, 11.2 mg sodium. Each serving of dumpling provides 43 calories, 2.3 g protein, 1 g saturated fat, 2 g unsaturated fat, 15 mg sodium.

---

# Pumpkin Soup

Pumpkin is a gold mine of beta-carotene, an important antioxidant shown to lower the risk of many cancers, especially lung, stomach, and prostate. Pumpkin also provides heart-healthy potassium and magnesium and is very low in sodium and calories. A weight watcher's delight! The sunflower seeds add a delicious crunch and the antioxidant vitamin E.

½ cup minced onion
1 tablespoon chicken fat or olive oil
3 cups chicken or vegetable stock
3 cups pumpkin puree
¼ teaspoon freshly grated pepper

¼ teaspoon freshly grated nutmeg,
   or to taste
Toasted sunflower seeds or toasted
   sliced almonds for garnish

In a heavy bottom saucepan, sauté onion in chicken fat or oil until golden but not brown. Add the stock, pumpkin puree, and seasonings and heat. Serve with toasted seeds or nuts.

*Yield:* 6 servings

---

**Each serving provides approximately 50 calories, 2 g protein, 2.25 g unsaturated fat, 5 mg sodium.**

---

# Sweet Potato, Banana, and Apricot Soup with Toasted Almond Garnish

Sweet potatoes (or pumpkin or squash as a substitute) are wonderful sources of the antioxidants beta-carotene, vitamin A, and vitamin C. They also provide potassium, calcium, and magnesium.

6 dried apricots

1 cup orange or apple juice

3 cups sweet potatoes, scrubbed and cut into chunks

1 cup sliced leeks or onions

1 cup scrubbed and chunked carrots

2 large stalks celery, including tops, sliced

1 large or 2 small shallots, chopped

1 medium banana

1 tablespoon grated orange rind

½ teaspoon cinnamon

Freshly grated nutmeg to taste

Freshly ground pepper to taste (optional)

1 cup of milk or light cream

2 tablespoons oat bran or wheat germ

Toasted chopped almonds for garnish

Soak the apricots in the fruit juice for 2 hours or overnight. Or place them in a 2-cup glass measure with 2 tablespoons of juice. Cover with plastic wrap and microcook for 2 minutes. Do not drain.

Place the sweet potatoes, leeks or onions, carrots, celery, and shallot in steamer basket (do not allow vegetables to touch the water), and steam until soft.

Transfer the vegetables to a food processor fitted with the steel blade. Add the apricots with the juice, the banana, orange rind, cinnamon, nutmeg, pepper, milk or light cream, and oat bran. Process until smooth. Check seasoning. Pour into bowls and garnish with toasted almonds.

## MICROWAVE METHOD

Instead of steaming the vegetables, place them in a 9-inch glass pie plate. Cover tightly with microwave plastic wrap and microcook for 6 minutes. Then proceed as above.

*Yield:* 6 servings

---

**Each serving provides 200 calories, 6 g protein, 2 g fat, just a trace of sodium.**

---

# Creamy Apricot-Carrot Soup

This soup delights your taste buds and nourishes your body. The pectin in the apricots has been shown to inhibit colon cancer; the very high concentration of beta-carotene (923 IU in one fresh apricot) has been shown to block cancer formation, especially of the lung and skin and others linked to cigarette smoking. Carrots, of course, are king of the beta-carotene family (7,930 IU in one medium carrot).

When you get a partnership of apricots and carrots, as you do in this delicious soup, you've got a powerful anticancer force working for you.

2 tablespoons butter or canola oil
½ cup chopped onion
1 stalk celery, chopped
2 cups carrots, scrubbed or pared
   and sliced
2 cups vegetable broth

8 dried apricots
1 cup milk
1 teaspoon Salt-Free Herbal
   Seasoning (page 143)
¼ teaspoon nutmeg
⅛ teaspoon freshly grated pepper

In a 2-quart saucepan, warm the butter or oil and add onion and celery. Cook until tender, but not brown. Add the sliced carrots and cook 5 minutes.

Add the broth and the apricots. Bring to a boil. Cover the pot and cook over medium heat 20 minutes, or until carrots are tender.

Puree in blender or food processor. Pour in saucepan, add milk, seasoning, nutmeg, and pepper. Simmer for 5 minutes but do not boil. Serve immediately.

*Yield:* 5 servings

---

**Each serving provides 127 calories, 3.1 g protein, 3.2 g saturated fat; 2 g unsaturated fat, 46 mg sodium.**

---

# Cream of Broccoli Soup

One of the easiest ways to sneak vitamin C–rich broccoli into a child's (or grown-up's) diet is to puree it with flavorful broth and some cream.

1 large head broccoli, washed and
    cut into florets
2 tablespoons minced onion
2 stalks celery, sliced
2 tablespoons butter

¼ cup soy flour
4 cups water or vegetable broth
2 cups milk or light cream or half
    of each
Dash of freshly grated nutmeg

Steam the broccoli or cook in a small amount of boiling water just until crisp-tender. Whiz in a blender or food processor until pureed.

Sauté onion and celery in the butter. Blend in the flour, then stir in the water or broth. Cook, stirring, until slightly thickened. Stir in broccoli, cream or milk, and nutmeg.

## MICROWAVE METHOD

In a 2½-quart soufflé dish, microcook the onion, celery, and butter, uncovered, on full power for 1½ minutes, or until onion is softened but not brown. Stir in the broccoli. Microcook, covered, on full power for 2 to 3 minutes or until broccoli is tender. Substitute 2 tablespoons of cornstarch for the soy flour, and stir it in. Add the water or broth and mix well. Microcook, uncovered, on full power for 3 to 4 minutes or until the mixture is thickened and bubbly, stirring twice. Combine the hot broccoli mixture and cream or milk in food processor and process until the mixture is nearly smooth. Pour back into the soufflé dish and microcook, uncovered, on full power for 1 minute or until the mixture is heated through. Do not boil. Garnish with grated nutmeg.

*Yield:* 6 servings

---

**Each serving provides approximately 109 calories, 5 g protein, 3.4 g saturated fat, 3 g unsaturated fat, 47 mg sodium.**

---

# Mushroom-Barley Soup

Few foods say "welcome home" more warmly than a rich barley-and-mushroom soup, simmering on your stove.

| | |
|---|---|
| ½ cup raw barley | 1 tablespoon oil or butter |
| 4 cups water or stock | ½ pound fresh mushrooms, sliced |
| 1 large bay leaf | 1 teaspoon dried thyme |
| 2 carrots, sliced | 1 tablespoon reduced-sodium |
| 1 small parsnip, sliced | soy sauce |
| ½ cup chopped onion | White pepper to taste |
| ½ teaspoon chopped garlic | ½ cup chopped fresh parsley |

In a large soup pot, simmer the barley in water or stock with the bay leaf, until barley is soft, about 1 hour. Add the carrots and parsnip, and simmer 15 minutes longer.

In a separate skillet, gently sauté the onion and garlic in the oil or butter until wilted. Add the mushrooms and thyme. Cook until soft, then add all the vegetables to the pot of barley. Add the soy sauce and pepper and bring to a boil.

Turn off the heat and let it stand 5 minutes before serving in order to blend the flavors. Sprinkle with chopped parsley and ladle into preheated bowls. This soup reheats beautifully but expect it to thicken.

*Yield:* 6 bowls

---

**Each bowl provides approximately 73 calories, 2 g protein, 1.5 g unsaturated fat, 53 mg sodium.**

---

*Variations:* You can transform this soup into a stew by adding $^1/_2$ cup of lentils and sliced celery to the stock pot 45 minutes before the barley is done.

To make the classic hearty Scotch Broth, simply add bits and pieces of lamb and bones to the above recipe.

---

### THE FIBER FILE

Bear in mind that leaving the skin on fruits and vegetables (potatoes, apples, pears, cucumbers, carrots) greatly increases fiber content.

When it comes to soluble fiber, however, it's the *bean family* that stands out. Beans of all kinds are better tasting and less expensive than oat bran when it comes to lowering cholesterol levels. As little as a half cup of cooked beans has the same amount of soluble fiber as $^2/_3$ cup of oat bran.

How can you increase your intake of beans? Add some lentils, kidney beans, chick-peas, split peas, pintos, mung beans, limas, or any of the colorful members of the bean family to a meat dish or to a soup and you will boost the nutritional wallop of that dish. It's a very good idea—health-wise, budget-wise, weight-wise, and cholesterol-wise to use less meat and more beans to bridge the gap.

Store uncooked dried beans in tightly covered glass jars. Stored in a cool, dry place, beans will keep for months. A few bay leaves in each container discourage insects.

Cook beans in a heavy pot, cast iron enamelware, unglazed pottery, or heavy-bottomed stainless steel.

Since preparing dried beans is a lengthy procedure, cook the beans you want now and for some future meals all at once. Beans freeze well and keep in the freezer for as long as five months. Freeze the extra beans in several separate containers that you can defrost as needed. Date the containers. Most beans keep their shape and texture nicely.

Keep a jar of cooked, marinated beans in the refrigerator, and use them to add texture and zest to a green salad.

Use leftover bean dishes as a stuffing base for peppers or cabbage or eggplant, or mix them with fresh vegetables in casseroles.

Add cooked beans to stir-fries.

Add sprouted mung and adzuki beans to your fresh vegetable salads.

Sprout garbanzos. Add them to salads, soups, stews, or stir-fries.

Bean flour can be added to baked goods to boost fiber and nutrition. You can make bean flour by grinding any kind of dried bean very finely. Or you can purchase soy and garbanzo flours at natural food stores. For every cup of flour called for in a recipe, substitute 2 or 3 tablespoons of bean flour for an equal amount of the wheat flour. This will enhance the quality of the protein because beans and grains contain complementary proteins.

Beans are not just for soups, stews, and salads. They are fantastic in baked goods. See, for example, the recipe for Bean Muffins.

# Lentil-Potato Soup

The wonderful aroma of this soup explains perfectly why Esau could not resist selling his birthright for a bowl of its rich hearty goodness. Lentils are a good source of many important minerals like calcium, magnesium, and potassium. Next to soy, they provide more protein than any other member of the legume family. Leave the skins on potatoes whenever possible—they provide protease inhibitors, which tend to block free-radical activity.

½ cup red lentils
3 medium-size potatoes (about 1 pound), scrubbed but unpeeled and diced
2 large onions, peeled and diced (about 2½ cups)
2 bay leaves
½ teaspoon no-salt vegetable seasoning, or to taste
¼ teaspoon dill weed

¼ teaspoon freshly grated pepper
6 cups water, chicken, or vegetable stock
2 tablespoons lecithin granules
2 tablespoons oat bran
1 hard-cooked egg, peeled and sliced (optional)
¼ cup chopped fresh parsley
Yogurt

In a large soup pot, bring lentils, potatoes, onions, all the seasonings, and water, chicken, or vegetable stock to a boil over high heat. Reduce heat to moderate and simmer for 1 hour, until lentils are very tender.

Process the soup, in 2 batches, in the food processor. Pour soup back into the pot, add the lecithin and oat bran and another ½ cup of water or stock if the soup is too thick.

To serve, top each bowl of soup with egg slices, parsley, and a dollop of yogurt.

*Yield:* Six 1-cup servings

**Each serving provides approximately 147 calories, 7 g protein, 1.5 g fat, 19 mg sodium.**

# Jacob's Lentil Stew

A snap to prepare, this lentil stew is made from ingredients you are likely to have on hand. Lentils are a nutritionist's dream because they supply impressive doses of dietary fiber, protein, and complex carbohydrates.

1 cup lentils

4 cups water or vegetable stock

1 large onion, coarsely chopped

2 cloves garlic, minced

3 carrots, sliced

1 teaspoon Salt-Free Herbal
  Seasoning (page 143)

2 teaspoons lemon juice

1 cup diced, unpeeled, potato

Wash lentils and place in a large pot with water or stock. Cook 30 minutes, then add remaining ingredients. Cook until vegetables are fork-tender.

*Yield:* 6 servings

Each serving provides 151 calories, 9 g protein, an insignificant amount of fat, 26 mg sodium.

## MICROWAVE INSTRUCTIONS

Combine lentils, onion, and water or stock in a large microsafe bowl. Microcook on high for 15 minutes. Add the remaining ingredients and microcook on high for an additional 10 minutes or until vegetables are fork tender.

### LENTILS—OF BIBLICAL FAME

According to grain expert Rebecca Wood, lentils are one of the world's first cultivated crops, eaten throughout the world as an inexpensive source of protein, and dubbed as "the poor man's meat" (*The Whole Foods Encyclopedia,* Prentice-Hall).

Like other members of the legume family, lentils are a fine source of fiber, both soluble and insoluble, and are low in fat and calories.

Here's another compelling reason to make them part of your diet: According to Earl Mindell, R.P.H., Ph.D., "lentils contain phytates which appear to help ward off cancerous changes in cells" (*Food as Medicine*, Simon and Schuster). The lentil recipes that appear here will help to reinforce your cancer resistance.

# Hearty Black- and Soybean Soup

Beans are a wonderful source of soluble fiber. The soybeans provide genistein, an important anticancer nutrient. The garlic, carrot, celery, and lemon contribute delightful taste accents along with anticancer phytochemicals. The potato and especially its skin provides chlorogenic acid, which has been shown to nip precancer cells in the bud.

| | |
|---|---|
| 1 cup black turtle beans, or black-eyed peas | 1 carrot |
| ½ cup soybeans | 1 bay leaf |
| 1½ quarts water or vegetable stock | 1 teaspoon dried oregano |
| 2 tablespoons canola or olive oil | 2 teaspoons no-salt vegetable seasoning |
| 1 medium onion, chopped | ⅛ teaspoon pepper |
| 1 clove garlic, crushed | Juice of 1 lemon |
| 2 stalks celery with leaves | ½ lemon, thinly sliced |
| 1 potato, scrubbed but unpeeled | |

Wash the beans and put them in a large saucepan with the water or stock and 1 tablespoon oil. Cover and bring to a boil, then simmer for about 2 hours, or until beans are almost tender.

Sauté the onion in the remaining oil with garlic until soft. Chop the celery, including the leaves. Grate potato and carrot coarsely. Add celery, potato, and carrot to onion and cook over medium heat for several minutes, stirring constantly.

Add the vegetables and seasonings to the beans in the last hour of their cooking. Bring the soup to a boil and lower heat to simmer until the beans and vegetables are done. Puree half or all the soup, if you desire. Add lemon juice and garnish with lemon slices just before serving.

**Yield:** Nine 1-cup servings

---

**Each serving provides approximately 150 calories, 11 g protein, 1 g saturated fat, 1.5 g unsaturated fat, 11 mg sodium.**

---

# Spinach and Cornmeal Soup

Popeye would flex his biceps for this soup. Both cornmeal and spinach are good muscle-building foods. Spinach is high in vitamin A, potassium, and iron and is very high in chlorophyll, a substance that has been shown to be a key anticancer agent. It is very low in calories. Cornmeal provides protein, trace minerals, and all the important B vitamins.

| | |
|---|---|
| 1 pound fresh spinach, or 1 package of frozen, chopped spinach | Freshly ground black pepper to taste |
| 1 tablespoon butter | ½ teaspoon freshly grated nutmeg |
| 1 tablespoon olive oil | ½ cup yellow cornmeal |
| 1 clove garlic | ¼ cup soy flour |
| 4 cups vegetable or chicken broth or water | Freshly popped corn (optional), or toasted sunflower seeds |

If you're using fresh spinach, wash it several times in lukewarm water. Steam or cook the spinach for about 8 minutes, using only the water that clings to the leaves. Chop the cooked spinach or process it for about 10 seconds in the food processor.

Heat the butter and oil in a pot, add garlic. When the garlic turns golden, remove and discard it.

Add the spinach and broth to the butter-oil mixture. Simmer over low heat for 3 minutes, then add pepper to taste and nutmeg.

In a small bowl, mix together the cornmeal and soy flour. Add ½ cup of the broth and stir vigorously until there are no lumps. Add this mixture to the soup pot and stir until soup is smooth.

Simmer over very low heat for 30 minutes. Garnish with popcorn or sunflower seeds.

## MICROWAVE METHOD

In a 2½-quart soufflé dish, microcook the butter, oil, and garlic, uncovered, for about 2 minutes, or until garlic is golden. Discard garlic and add the cleaned spinach. Microcook, covered, on full power for 2 minutes. Mix the cornmeal and flour. Add ½ cup of the broth to the cornmeal and flour mixture, and stir to prevent lumps. Blend this into the rest of the broth. Add the pepper to taste and nutmeg. Add this mixture to the soufflé dish and microcook, covered, on full power for about 6 minutes.

*Yield:* 6 servings

---

**Each serving provides 70 calories, 3 g protein, 1.2 g saturated fat, 3 g unsaturated fat, 8 mg sodium.**

# Cream of Chestnut Soup

Every time I sip this soup, all of my senses are pleasantly stimulated. So flavorful, it works miracles on those in grumpy moods. Chestnuts have all the rich hearty flavor of the nut family without the high fat content.

| | |
|---|---|
| 1 pound chestnuts (in the shell) | 2 cups vegetable or chicken stock |
| 1 medium onion, diced | 1 teaspoon honey |
| 2 tablespoons olive oil | ¾ cup light cream or evaporated |
| 1 medium carrot | skim milk |

With a sharp knife, cut an × in the flat side of each chestnut. Cover with water and boil 15 minutes, then peel as soon as they are cool enough to handle.

Heat the oil and sauté the onion for about 2 minutes or until lightly browned. Scrub the carrot and cut into ½-inch slices. Add the onion and carrot to the chestnuts. Add the vegetable or chicken stock and bring to a boil. Reduce heat and simmer until chestnuts are soft, about 15 minutes. Pour liquid through a colander and reserve it. Puree the chestnut mixture in the food processor. Return to the liquid and heat. Combine the honey and the cream or milk and add to the chestnut mixture. Heat but do not boil. This soup can also be served at room temperature or chilled. Delicious at any temperature.

## MICROWAVE METHOD

Cut chestnuts as above. Combine with ½ cup water in a shallow dish, uncovered, and microcook on full power for 8 minutes. Peel when they are cool enough to handle.

In a 2½-quart soufflé dish, microcook the onion in the olive oil, uncovered, for 2 minutes. Add the carrot, sliced thin, and microcook, covered, for 3 minutes. Add the vegetable or chicken stock and the peeled chestnuts and microcook, covered, for 6 minutes.

Transfer the mixture to a food processor and whiz until smooth. Return to soufflé dish, add the honey combined with the cream or milk, and microcook, covered, for about 2 minutes to reheat.

*Yield:* Six ¹/₂-cup servings

---

**Each serving provides 200 calories, 4 g protein, .6 g saturated fat, 7 g unsaturated fat, just a trace of soduim.**

---

# Squash and Tahini Soup

You've got to taste this soup to believe its smooth, rich, delicate flavor. It's love at first sip. In fact, tahini is one of the ingredients used by Egyptian women in ancient times to enhance their love life. Tahini is made from sesame seeds which are 45 percent protein and very rich in polyunsaturated fat—the "good" fat that won't clog your arteries. I'm not vouching for what they'll do to your love life, but watch out!

| | |
|---|---|
| 1 tablespoon olive oil | ⅛ teaspoon ground cloves |
| 2 tablespoons finely chopped onion | ½ teaspoon honey |
| 2 cups cooked squash or pumpkin | 1 teaspoon lemon juice |
| 2½ cups stock or water | 2 tablespoons tahini |
| 2½ cups milk | Pumpkin seeds for garnish |

In a heavy saucepan, heat the oil, add the onion, and cook for only 2 minutes, stirring, until they are transparent. Add the squash, stock or water, milk, cloves, honey, and lemon juice. Stir thoroughly. Bring to a boil, then reduce heat and cook, stirring occasionally, for 15 minutes. Stir in the tahini. Puree the soup in the food processor, then return to saucepan to be heated through. Do not let it come to a boil. Serve hot garnished with pumpkin seeds. This soup is also excellent when served chilled with a dollop of yogurt or, if you want to be fancy, whipped cream.

## MICROWAVE METHOD

In a 2½-quart soufflé dish, microcook the oil and onion, uncovered, for 1 minute or until onion is transparent. Add the squash and microcook, covered, for 2 minutes. Puree the squash mixture in the food processor. Return to the soufflé dish and add the stock or water, milk, cloves, honey, lemon juice, and tahini. Cover and microwave on full power for 4 minutes.

*Yield:* 6 to 8 servings

---

**Each of 6 servings provides 87 calories, 4 g protein, 2 g fat. Each of 8 servings provides 65 calories, 3 g protein, 1 g fat, just a trace of sodium.**

---

# Chilled Strawberry Soup in Melon Bowls

A soup like this says "love" in the most delicious way. Besides being a feast for the eyes, it provides many of the nutrients that hearty warm soups provide, but without the heat. Both strawberries and melons provide many minerals and vitamins C and A. Cantaloupe is extraordinarily rich in carotene too.

Strawberries, besides their luscious flavor, have high concentrations of ellagic acid, a potent anticancer agent. Enjoy this soup and increase your chances of staying young and healthy longer!

1 quart fresh strawberries, washed
    and hulled
1 cup orange juice
1¼ teaspoons instant tapioca
⅛ teaspoon ground allspice
⅛ teaspoon cinnamon

2 tablespoons honey
1 teaspoon grated lemon rind
1 tablespoon lemon juice, or to taste
1 cup buttermilk or yogurt
2 chilled cantaloupes or honeydew
    melons

Set aside 8 strawberries. Puree remaining berries in blender or food processor. Strain into saucepan. Add orange juice.

In a small bowl, mix tapioca with 4 tablespoons of pureed strawberry mixture. Add to saucepan along with remaining juice and berry mixture, allspice, and cinnamon.

Heat, stirring constantly, until mixture comes to a boil. Cook 1 minute or until thickened. Remove from heat. Pour soup into a large bowl or soup tureen. Add honey, lemon rind and juice, and buttermilk or yogurt, and blend well. Slice reserved berries and fold into soup. Cover and chill at least 8 hours.

Cut melons in half. Scoop out seeds. Turn upside down on paper towels to drain. Fill melons with luscious strawberry soup.

*Yield:* 4 servings

---

**Each serving provides approximately 194 calories, 5 g protein, insignificant fat and sodium.**

---

# Turkey Noodle Soup

This flavorful soup is the answer to everyone's fondest wish—a delicious soup that tastes as if it has simmered for hours, but is ready in less than a half hour. What's more, it's a great way to use your leftover turkey.

4 cups chicken or vegetable broth
2 cups diced cooked turkey or
   chicken
3 cloves garlic, minced
1 cup frozen mixed vegetables, or
   ½ cup each of sliced carrots and
   broccoli florets

1½ cups dry egg noodles
   (any style)
½ teaspoon vegetable seasoning or
   kelp
⅛ teaspoon freshly ground pepper
⅛ teaspoon ground sage

Combine all ingredients in a 3-quart glass bowl. Microwave on high for 12 minutes or until boiling. Stir. Microwave at medium for 15 minutes or until noodles are tender.

*Yield:* 6 hearty servings

---

**Each serving provides approximately 176 calories, 18 g protein, 2 g saturated fat, 3 g unsaturated fat, 506 mg sodium.**

---

# VEGETARIAN MAIN COURSES

According to statistics, vegetarians are healthier, more slender, and live longer than meat eaters. Why?

Because vegetarians eat more fruit, vegetables, nuts, seeds, and grains, which increases their consumption of a wide variety of life-saving antioxidants while reducing their intake of calories and saturated fats.

The word *vegetarian* does not, as one might infer, derive from vegetable. It is from the Latin *vegetus,* which means "whole, sound, fresh, lively."

Whether you are an ethical vegetarian or a meat eater seeking to reduce meat consumption, be assured that it is possible to maintain a sound, healthy, vigorous physical state on a vegetarian regimen—but you should have a rudimentary knowledge of protein patterns.

Eggs, meat, fish, and dairy products are complete proteins, which means they contain all the amino acids your body needs in the *correct proportions.* Because amino acids depend on one another to make body tissue, if one is absent, none can be utilized. It's like trying to make bricks without straw.

So, what's the formula? Here's a simple guide to use suggested by Dr. Robert J. Williams, author of *Nutrition Against Disease*: "Don't restrict yourself to one part of an organism. In the plant world, do not restrict yourself to green leaves, or to root vegetables, or to seeds or to fruits. Each of these is in itself incomplete."

## A VEGETARIAN HELPFUL HINT

Nuts, seeds, avocadoes, whole grains, and legumes are incomplete. But, according to Dr. Williams's formula, when eaten with raw green leafy vegetables, they provide complete protein, well utilized by the body.

The recipes in this chapter provide good protein patterns. But do enhance them and increase the pleasure of each meal with a fresh green salad.

# Garlicky Broccoli and Zucchini Pasta

A delicious way to reduce your cancer risk!

1 head broccoli, separated into florets

1 package (8 ounces) angel hair spaghetti or other pasta

2 tablespoons olive or canola oil

5 cloves garlic, minced

1 zucchini, cut into ½-inch cubes

1 teaspoon dried oregano

Salt-Free Herbal Seasoning (page 143) and freshly ground pepper to taste

1 tablespoon unsalted butter

½ cup freshly grated Parmesan cheese

½ cup sesame or sunflower seeds

Steam broccoli in a small amount of water or vegetable broth until crisp-tender (about 7 minutes).

Cook spaghetti according to package directions.

In a skillet or a wok, heat the oil and stir-fry the garlic and zucchini until zucchini is barely tender. Add oregano and seasonings to taste. Melt butter into sauce, then add broccoli.

Toss sauce with spaghetti and sprinkle with Parmesan and seeds.

*Yield:* 4 servings

---

**Each serving provides approximately 130 calories, 4 g protein, 3 g saturated fat, 4 g unsaturated fat, 44 mg sodium.**

---

# Tofu Manicotti

Recent research reveals that soybeans, from which tofu is derived, may play an important role in our fight against two deadly diseases: cancer and heart disease. The spotlight is on a compound called genistein, found only in the soybean family.

Green leafy vegetables, like spinach, provide many different kinds of carotenoids, and each offers protection from cancer. In this dish, you get all this and several more contenders for high honors in the anticancer limelight, namely garlic, onion, and tomato sauce.

½ pound fresh spinach
¼ cup minced onion
1 tablespoon canola or olive oil
2 pounds tofu
3 cloves garlic, pressed
2 tablespoons chopped fresh parsley
1 teaspoon Salt-Free Herbal
 Seasoning (page 143)

¼ teaspoon freshly ground
 pepper
Pinch of freshly grated nutmeg
Manicotti shells (preferably whole
 wheat)
Tomato sauce (canned or
 homemade)

Cook the spinach in water briefly, drain, and puree in blender or food processor. Sauté onion in the oil. Combine the spinach, onion, tofu, garlic, parsley, and seasonings, mashing until well mixed.

Prepare the manicotti for stuffing according to package instructions. Cool slightly. Stuff the manicotti shells with the tofu mixture.

Preheat oven to 350°F.

In an ovenproof casserole, layer the bottom with the tomato sauce, then add a layer of stuffed shells, then another layer of tomato sauce. Cover and bake for 40 minutes.

*Yield:* 4 servings

**Each serving provides 474 calories, 16 g protein, .5 g saturated fat, 5.5 g unsaturated fat, 38 mg sodium.**

# Betty's Zippy Pasta with Radish and Orange

Radishes and oranges may seem like an unusual combination, but the bite of radishes and sweetness of the oranges burst with flavor in your mouth.

| | |
|---|---|
| 8 ounces (3 cups) uncooked rotelle pasta | 2 tablespoons olive oil |
| 2 cups fresh spinach leaves in bite-size pieces | 2 tablespoons red wine vinegar |
| | 3 tablespoons plain yogurt |
| 1½ cups thinly sliced radishes | 1 teaspoon minced garlic |
| 1 cup fresh orange chunks | 1 teaspoon oregano leaves, crushed |
| | ½ teaspoon vegetable seasoning |

Cook pasta according to package directions. Drain and rinse under cool water. Place in a large bowl along with spinach, radishes, and orange chunks.

In a small bowl combine oil, vinegar, yogurt, garlic, oregano, and seasoning. Pour over the pasta mixture. Serve immediately or cover and refrigerate.

*Yield:* 7 cups, about 6 portions

---

**Each portion provides 322 calories, 10.3 g protein, .6 g saturated fat, 4.7 g unsaturated fat, 15 mg sodium.**

---

•◆•

## RADISHES

Don't underestimate the anticancer power in those little red fireballs you add to your salads for flavor, crunch, and color.

A relative of the mustard family and a member of the cruciferous family, a radish contains many of the same cancer-fighting compounds as its cousins, mustard greens, cabbage, and broccoli.

In particular, radishes contain isothiocyanates, which wield a double wallop against cancer. First, they perform like goaltenders: should a cancer-causing substance dare to invade your body, the isothiocyanates run interference and prevent the linkup. But that's not all. Should there be an existing cancer, they attack the supply line that is fueling it, and then suppress its growth.

Radishes act as bodyguards on other vital fronts: they are a weight and cholesterol watcher's crunchy delight. They are fat free, very low in sodium, a good source of vitamin C, potassium, and other trace minerals, and very low in calories. Enjoy seven radishes and you've consumed only 20 calories! What a bargain!

At the market, look for firm, crisp radishes with bright fresh greens (if still attached). Remove the greens because they tend to dehydrate the root radish. Radish greens add flavor and nutrition to soups and salads.

Perhaps you have never considered cooking with radishes. If so, you are about to discover a whole new world of culinary delights!

———————— •◆• ————————

# Butternut Squash Casserole

Squash is one of the deep orange vegetables very rich in anticancer nutrients. This easy to prepare and versatile dish can be served hot or cold, as a main dish for a heart-healthy meatless meal, or as a side dish for an elegant dinner party or a take-along buffet.

5 cups grated squash (about 1 pound)
Juice and grated rind of 1 lemon
1 cup raisins
10 dried apricots, diced
½ cup chopped prunes
1 large apple, washed and diced

1½ cups cottage cheese, drained
3 tablespoons plain yogurt
2 teaspoons cinnamon
⅛ teaspoon freshly grated nutmeg
1 egg
½ cup chopped walnuts

Combine the squash with the lemon juice and rind. Spread 3 cups of this mixture in a 9-by-12-by-2-inch casserole, buttered or coated with nonstick cooking spray.

Preheat oven to 375°F.

In a small bowl, combine the raisins, apricots, prunes, and apple. Spread this mixture over the squash.

Combine the cottage cheese, yogurt, cinnamon, nutmeg, and egg. Spread this mixture over the fruit mixture, then top with the remaining squash mixture. Sprinkle with chopped walnuts and bake for 30 minutes, or until deliciously golden.

*Yield:* 8 servings as a main dish, 16 servings as a side dish

---

**Each serving as a main dish provides approximately 227 calories, 11.3 g protein, .25 g saturated fat, 4.5 g unsaturated fat, 97 mg sodium.**

---

# Pumpkin Seed–Potato Cakes

Pumpkin seeds are full of potent cancer fighters, and they're also a good source of the mineral zinc.

If your sense of taste and smell have diminished, you may need more zinc. Sunflower seeds, sesame seeds, and pumpkin seeds are excellent sources of zinc.

Serve a dish of mixed seeds and raisins for dessert and TV snacks. Include seeds in your baking and stir-fries.

|  |  |
|---|---|
| 1 cup chopped pumpkin seeds | ¼ teaspoon freshly ground pepper |
| 2 cups seasoned mashed potatoes | ¼ cup wheat germ |
| 2 tablespoons chopped parsley | 2 tablespoons soy flour or powder |
| 1 egg, beaten | 1 tablespoon canola or olive oil |

Combine the chopped pumpkin seeds with the mashed potatoes and parsley. Add half the beaten egg and the pepper.

Combine the wheat germ and soy flour or powder.

Heat oil in a large nonstick frying pan.

Shape the seed mixture into 8 flat cakes. Dip cakes in the remaining egg, then in wheat germ mixture. Brown lightly on both sides. Have a lovely evening.

*Yield:* 4 servings

---

Each serving provides approximately 331 calories, 16 g protein, 4.2 g saturated fat, 14 g unsaturated fat, 38 mg sodium.

---

## PUMPKIN AND SQUASH

Rich in nutrients, low in calories, pumpkin and squash can embellish your meals from soup to dessert!

Nature is indeed wise and bountiful. Just when the leaves have rustled their last colorful hurrah and fresh garden produce has all but disappeared from the marketplace, we are offered a proliferation of vivid pumpkins and multihued squashes. Their bright colors and seductive shapes beg us to enjoy some now and store some for the cold time when we have an increased need for their many nutritional benefits.

Squash and pumpkin, cousins under the skin, are both gold mines of beta-carotene, an important antioxidant shown to inhibit the growth of tumors, and are so low in calories, they have been hailed as a weight-watcher's delight. And you get as much as 9,360 units of beta-carotene in 1 cup of squash, and a whopping 15,680 units in every cup of pumpkin.

That same cup of pumpkin also provides more potassium than you'd get in a large banana. You also benefit from the B vitamins, calcium, iron, some vitamin C, and 2.5 grams of protein in every cup. All this and just 81 calories! What a bonanza, especially for those who wish to stay slim or lose weight and feel great.

A very easy way to prepare a great big winter squash is simply to bake it. Cut it into servings about 4 inches square. Lay these pieces on a lightly oiled cookie sheet, skin side down, Brush with oil, season with cinnamon, nutmeg, or mace. Bake until tender and serve as is, or use in any recipe that calls for cooked squash or pumpkin. If you have more than you can use right away, bake some until it is not quite tender and freeze.

You can also enhance the taste and nutritional benefits of any soup simply by adding peeled and seeded winter squash. In vegetable or chicken broth, add savory herbs and puree to make a delicious, full-bodied soup.

---

# Almond and Cashew Loaf

My friend, Beatrice Trum Hunter, who was heavily involved in the natural foods movement in the early 1960s, created this recipe for her book, *The Natural Foods Cookbook*.

Though it is a vegetarian dish, it looks and tastes like meat loaf. For a real treat, try it with spaghetti sauce or salsa, or shape the mixture into patties instead of a loaf.

Hint: Always use unsalted nuts.

½ cup cashews, ground
½ cup almonds, ground
1 cup cooked brown rice
¼ cup soy grits, presoaked in ½ cup vegetable broth
1 egg, lightly beaten

1 large or 2 small onions, grated
¼ cup minced parsley
¼ cup wheat germ
½ teaspoon vegetable seasoning
½ teaspoon thyme

In a bowl, combine all ingredients and blend. Turn into an 8-by-4-inch loaf plan, oiled or spritzed with nonstick cooking spray. Bake at 350 °F for 30 minutes.

*Yield:* 8 servings

---

**Each serving provides approximately 152 calories, 8 g protein, 14 g saturated fat, 15 g unsaturated fat, 49 mg sodium.**

---

# Bean Burgers

A mouthful of guardian angels. That's how my grandkids describe these burgers. And why not? This bean burger is high in fiber, very tasty, and far preferable to its counterpart in the beef family. The combination of beans, sunflower seeds, wheat germ, and soy granules make it not only a complete protein but a dynamite team of antioxidants to protect many areas of your body from incipient malignancies. And they're so easy to make.

2 cups cooked beans, preferably kidney or fava
½ cup sunflower seeds
¼ cup chopped onion
½ teaspoon chili powder
2 tablespoons olive oil

3 to 4 tablespoons tomato sauce or catsup
¼ cup wheat germ
¼ cup soy grits or powder
8 thin slices low-fat mozzarella or Cheddar cheese (optional)

In a food processor blend together the beans, seeds, onion, and chili powder until smooth. Add the oil, tomato sauce or catsup, wheat germ, and soy granules. Process until ingredients are well combined.

Preheat oven to 350°F.

Form mixture into small patties. Place on lightly oiled baking sheet and bake for 15 to 20 minutes, or until lightly browned and crusty.

*Yield:* 4 servings of 2 burgers each

---

Each burger without cheese provides 125 calories, 8 g protein, 2 g saturated fat, 4.6 g unsaturated fat, just a trace of sodium.

---

# Sprouted Wheat and Nut Patties

Sprouting the wheat multiplies its antioxidant potential, making this combination of protease inhibitors a powerhouse anticancer duo.

2 cups wheat berry sprouts
½ cup peanuts, ground or chopped fine
½ cup pumpkin seeds
1 onion, grated
1 cup vegetable stock

2 tablespoons soy flour
1 teaspoon vegetable seasoning
2 tablespoons wheat germ
1 egg
2 cups whole-grain bread crumbs

Combine all ingredients except the bread crumbs in blender or food processor. Add enough bread crumbs to make mixture pliable enough to be shaped into patties. Arrange patties on an oiled cookie sheet. Broil on each side until temptingly brown.

*Yield:* 8 servings

---

Each serving provides approximately 185 calories, 9 g protein, 3.6 g saturated fat, 9.5 g unsaturated fat, 17 mg sodium.

---

# Brown Rice and Garbanzo Patties

Garbanzos are a rich source of protease inhibitors, valuable for their ability to shut down the cancer procress. Brown rice is a rich source of fiber and vitamin B and is also a protease inhibitor. The wheat germ provides vitamin E, a potent antioxidant, and the Brazil nuts provide selenium, the mineral antioxidant that works in tandem with vitamin E, enhancing the power of both. Put them all together and you've got preventive medicine in a delicious, crunchy patty.

2 cups cooked short-grain brown rice
1 cup cooked or sprouted garbanzos
¼ cup wheat germ
⅓ cup Brazil nuts
¼ cup vegetable stock

1 teaspoon onion powder
½ teaspoon celery seed
½ teaspoon Salt-Free Herbal
   Seasoning (page 143)
½ teaspoon cayenne

Combine all ingredients in a food processor and mince to a medium-fine grain. Shape into thin patties and place on a baking sheet sprayed with nonstick cooking spray. Place in a 375°F oven and bake until brown and crispy, about 30 minutes. Serve with cranberry, apple, or tomato sauce.

*Yield:* 6 servings

Each serving provides approximately 145 calories, 5 g protein, 4.2 g unsaturated fat, just a trace of sodium.

# Sunflower Patties

The sunflower seed is like a little sunlamp in your digestive system. It is one of the few foods that provide the vitamin D, so necessary to the utilization of calcium and phosphorus. Its high protein content (24 percent) makes it an excellent substitute for meat.

1 tablespoon canola or olive oil
3 tablespoons chopped onion
1 clove garlic, minced
½ cup finely chopped mushrooms
½ cup chopped celery, including leaves
½ cup grated carrots
2 tablespoons chopped green pepper
⅓ cup water or vegetable broth
1 egg
1 cup ground sunflower seeds

2 tablespoons wheat germ
2 tablespoons chopped fresh parsley, or 1 teaspoon dried
½ teaspoon kelp
¼ teaspoon dry mustard
1 teaspoon finely chopped fresh basil, or ½ teaspoon dried
2 teaspoons reduced-sodium Tamari soy sauce
¼ cup tomato sauce, or as much as needed to bind ingredients

In a large skillet, heat the oil and sauté the onion, garlic, mushrooms, celery, carrots, and pepper for 2 minutes. Add the water or broth, cover the skillet, and allow mixture to steam-sauté over medium heat for 3 minutes. Pour the mixture into a large bowl and add the remaining ingredients.

Preheat the oven to 350°F.

Mix the ingredients well. Form into patties about the size of hamburgers, arrange in an oiled shallow baking dish about 10-by-6 inches. Bake until brown—about 20 minutes. Turn and brown the other side—about 10 minutes.

*Yield:* 8 patties

**Each patty provides approximately 90 calories, 9.5 g protein, .5 g saturated fat, 2.5 g unsaturated fat, 30 mg sodium.**

*Variations:* 1. Coat with sesame seeds before baking.

2. Patties may be sautéed or broiled.

3. Try broiling with Cheddar cheese on top.

# Kasha and Sesame Seed Patties

A vegetarian burger that rivals the original in popularity. Kasha, or buchwheat groats, is a stick-to-your-ribs comfort food, high in fiber, very low in fat. It improves glucose tolerance, making it a great food for diabetics. Because it is a nonwheat member of the rhubarb family, it is also a great food for those allergic to wheat.

| | |
|---|---|
| 1 teaspoon canola or olive oil | 1 cup mushrooms, chopped |
| 1 medium-size onion, thinly sliced | 1 tablespoon chopped fresh parsley |
| 1 cup coarse-grain kasha (buckwheat groats), cooked | 2 tablespoons sesame seeds |
| | 2 eggs |

In a skillet, heat oil and lightly sauté onion and mushrooms for about 3 minutes. Add this mixture to the cooked kasha. In bowl or food processor, beat together the parsley, sesame seeds, and eggs and combine with the kasha.

Form into 3-inch patties and sauté on both sides in a hot oiled skillet or bake in a 350°F oven for about 10 minutes, or until crisp on the outside but still moist on the inside. Serve in warm rolls with mustard, hot tomato sauce, or pickled relish. Enjoy a vegetarian picnic.

*Yield:* 8 patties

**Each patty provides approximately 113 calories, 3.8 g protein, .3 g saturated fat, .8 g unsaturated fat, 17 mg sodium.**

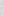 

# Lentil-Millet Loaf

The combination of lentils and millet makes this a nicely balanced and delicious meal—a favorite among vegetarians. Apple, carrot, and soy enhance the flavor and antioxidant and phytochemical value of this one-dish meal.

1½ cups cooked lentils (½ cup brown lentils and ½ teaspoon herbal seasoning, added to 1½ cups water and cooked for 30 minutes)

1 cup cooked millet (¼ cup millet and ¼ teaspoon herbal seasoning, added slowly to 1 cup boiling water and cooked over low heat for 30 minutes)

2 eggs

1 apple, well scrubbed, unpeeled

½ cup grated carrot

1 tablespoon sesame or canola oil

1 teaspoon kelp

½ teaspoon Salt-Free Herbal Seasoning (page 143)

½ teaspoon dried parsley or chives

2 tablespoons toasted sesame seeds

Combine all ingredients except the sesame seeds in mixing bowl or food processor and process briefly. Pour the mixture into a 9-by-5-inch loaf pan, lightly oiled or spritzed with a nonstick cooking spray. Sprinkle with the sesame seeds.

Preheat oven to 375°F.

Bake for 45 minutes in the oven or microwave, uncovered, on high for about 10 minutes.

*Yield:* 8 servings

---

**Each serving provides approximately 112 calories, 5.8 g protein, .7 g saturated fat, 3.3 g unsaturated fat, 9 mg sodium.**

# Luscious Vegetarian Lasagna

This dish is practically a prescription for preventive medicine. Enjoy it in good health!

1 cup chopped onions

3 cloves garlic, minced

2 cups diced zucchini

1½ cups sliced mushrooms

1 cup diced sweet green peppers

½ cup sliced carrots

1 cup broccoli florets

One 28-ounce can crushed tomatoes

1½ cups water or vegetable stock

One 8-ounce can tomato paste

1 tablespoon chopped fresh basil, or
   1 teaspoon dried

½ teaspoon crushed dried rosemary

½ teaspoon freshly ground black
   pepper

2 cups nonfat ricotta cheese

1½ cups shredded part-skim
   mozzarella cheese

8 ounces lasagna, cooked

In a 4-quart pot, coated with nonstick cooking spray, sauté the onions and garlic over medium-high heat for about 3 minutes, stirring frequently.

Add the zucchini, mushrooms, peppers, and carrots. Cook, stirring frequently, until vegetables are crisp-tender—about 6 minutes.

Stir in the tomatoes, water, tomato paste, and seasonings. Bring to a boil. Reduce the heat, cover the pot, and simmer for about 20 minutes. Set aside 2 cups of this sauce.

In a medium bowl, combine the ricotta and 1 cup of the mozzarella.

Preheat oven to 350°F.

In a 9-by-13-inch baking dish, spread one-third of the remaining sauce. Place one-third of the lasagna noodles over the sauce and spread half the cheese mixture over them. Repeat the layers. Top with the remaining third of the sauce and then the remaining third of the noodles. Then spread the remaining 2 cups of sauce over the noodles.

Cover the dish with foil and bake for 25 minutes. Remove the foil and sprinkle the remaining ½ cup of mozzarella over the lasagna. Bake until the cheese melts and the lasagna is bubbling hot.

*Yield:* 8 servings

Each serving provides approximately 250 calories, 6 g protein, 3 g saturated fat, 2 g unsaturated fat, 250 mg sodium.

# Asparagus Loaf

A loaf studded with gorgeous asparagus and so perfectly seasoned you'll never believe it has anticancer properties.

1 cup whole-grain bread cubes

2 tablespoons butter

1 tablespoons chopped parsley

1 teaspoon finely grated onion

½ teaspoon Salt-Free Herbal
    Seasoning (page 143)

2 eggs

2 cups hot milk

4 cups 1-inch pieces of
    asparagus

Preheat oven to 375°F.

In a skillet over medium heat sauté bread cubes in the butter with the parsley, onion, and herbal seasoning for about 5 minutes.

Beat eggs slightly, add a small amount of hot milk to the eggs, stirring constantly. Then blend slowly into the remaining hot milk.

Combine the milk mixture and the asparagus.

Bake in a loaf pan approximately 5½-by-9 inches for about 30 minutes, or until set.

*Yield:* 6 servings

Each serving provides approximately 159 calories, 70 g protein, 7 g saturated fat, 2 g unsaturated fat, 516 mg sodium.

### ASPARAGUS

Asparagus is a source of nutrients that spur the production of glutathione, an important antioxidant. Gluthathione has the power to engage and destroy toxins and neutralize carcinogens.

Besides the glutathione, asparagus provides lots of beta-carotene (1.31 IU in one cup), a goodly amount of B vitamins and vitamins C and E, as well as potassium and zinc.

When choosing asparagus, buy bright green spears with compact tips and use it as soon as possible. Store asparagus loosely covered in the refrigerator. To keep it fresh, wrap a moist paper towel around the stems or stand it upright in about two inches of cold water. Snap off the fibrous stalks and use for vegetable stock.

# Baked Asparagus and Mushroom Casserole

This tastes best if cooked a day in advance then reheated in the oven. It gives the flavors a chance to meld.

1 pound fresh asparagus, washed
   and trimmed
½ pound fresh mushrooms
2 tablespoons butter
   (optional)

¼ cup whole wheat flour
1 teaspoon vegetable seasoning
1 cup milk
¼ cup grated Cheddar cheese

Arrange the asparagus in a 9-by-11-inch baking pan. Preheat oven to 375°F. Wash and slice mushrooms and arrange them over the asparagus.

Prepare a béchamel sauce with the butter, flour, seasoning, and milk. Pour the sauce over the asparagus and mushrooms.

Cover and bake for about 20 minutes.

Uncover and sprinkle cheese over asparagus and mushroom mixture. Bake, uncovered, for 5 more minutes or until cheese is brown and bubbly.

*Yield:* 4 servings

---

Each serving provides approximately 136 calories, 10.3 g protein, 5 g saturated fat, 4.1 g unsaturated fat, 89 mg sodium.

---

# Tofu Chili

Tofu, a soy product that provides cancer-fighting genistein, substitutes for meat in this hearty chili.

| | |
|---|---|
| 2 pounds firm tofu | 1 teaspoon cumin |
| 2 tablespoons olive or canola oil | 1 tablespoon vinegar |
| 1 large onion, diced | 1 teaspoon honey |
| 2 cloves garlic, minced | 1 teaspoon Salt-Free Herbal |
| 4 cups cooked kidney beans | Seasoning (page 143) |
| 3 cups unpeeled, chopped tomatoes, (fresh or canned) | ¼ teaspoon freshly ground pepper |
| | Cayenne pepper to taste |
| 1 to 3 tablespoons chili powder, according to taste | |

Press the tofu and crumble it.

In a large pot or wok, heat the oil and sauté the onion and garlic until tender. Add tofu and sauté another few minutes. Add all remaining ingredients and simmer for 20 minutes.

*Yield:* 8 hearty servings

---

**Each serving provides approximately 255 calories, 29.6 g protein, 1 g saturated fat, 6 g unsaturated fat, 4.4 mg sodium.**

---

# Tofu Stir-fry with Walnuts

The walnuts contribute protease inhibitors, which tend to block cancer development before it gets to first base; also cancer-fighting polyphenols; a rich supply of omega-3 fatty acids; and a delightful texture contrast. The ginger contributes incredible flavor.

1 large onion, chopped
1 tablespoon sesame, olive, or
    canola oil
4 large mushrooms, sliced
1 cup 1-inch pieces of string beans
1 teaspoon powdered ginger
1 tablespoon finely chopped ginger
    root (optional)
1 large clove garlic, crushed

1½ tablespoons arrowroot powder
⅔ cup water
2 tablespoons reduced-sodium
    Tamari soy sauce
1 tablespoon wine or cider vinegar
1 teaspoon honey
1 pound tofu, cut into 1-inch cubes
½ cup chopped walnuts
Chopped fresh parley

In a heavy skillet or in a wok, sauté the onion in the oil over medium heat for 1 minute. Add the sliced mushrooms and string beans (any vegetable may be substituted). Cover the pan and steam for 5 minutes. Add the two kinds of ginger and the garlic. Combine the arrowroot and water and add to the pot. Add the soy sauce, vinegar, and honey.

Turn the heat up and stir vigorously as you bring the mixture to a boil. Then lower the heat to simmer and add the tofu and walnuts. Simmer for a few minutes, until the sauce thickens. Garnish with parsley. Serve as is or over cooked brown rice or cooked pasta. A delight to the eyes and the palate.

*Yield:* 4 servings

---

**Each serving provides approximately 231 calories, 6 g protein, 1 g saturated fat, 9 g unsaturated fat, 4 mg sodium.**

---

# Squash Casserole

A tasty and hearty main dish, sauced with yogurt, cottage cheese, and chives.

3 cups ¼-inch pieces of winter
    squash (butternut preferably)
½ cup chopped onions
½ cup shredded carrots
½ cup chopped celery

2 tablespoons butter
¾ cup whole wheat bread crumbs
½ teaspoon dried basil
½ teaspoon dried thyme
¼ teaspoon white pepper

### Sauce

1 cup plain yogurt
¼ cup grated mild cheese
1 egg, beaten
2 tablespoons chopped fresh chives or scallions
¼ cup toasted sesame seeds

Preheat the oven to 350°F.

Steam or microwave the squash until tender. Combine the vegetables and butter with the bread crumbs, then add the basil, thyme, and pepper, making a stuffing.

Make a layer of half the squash in the bottom of a greased 2-quart casserole. Place the stuffing on top, then the remaining squash.

### TO MAKE THE SAUCE

Stir the yogurt and grated cheese together. Place over low heat until the cheese melts. Stir a little of the sauce into the beaten egg, then add this mixture to the sauce slowly to prevent curdling. Add the chives or scallions. Pour the yogurt sauce over the squash casserole and sprinkle with toasted sesame seeds. Bake for 30 minutes.

*Yield:* 4 servings

---

Each serving with the sauce provides approximately 211 calories, 5 g protein, 3 g saturated fat, 3 g unsaturated fat, 168 mg sodium.

---

*Sauce yield:* 1 1/2 cups

---

Each 1/4 cup provides approximately 72 calories, 4 g protein, 1.5 g saturated fat, 2.5 g unsaturated fat, 109 mg sodium.

---

# Ratatouille with Almond

Almonds' high ration of monounsaturated fatty acids lowers LDLs, the bad cholesterol. When these nuts are combined with a powerful gang of antioxidants and phytochemical-rich foods like eggplant, zucchini, peppers, onion, garlic, and tomatoes, you've got a healthy, hearty, sumptuous meal with built-in cancer protection.

2 tablespoons olive or canola oil

2 cloves garlic, crushed

1 large onion, thinly sliced

1 small eggplant, cubed

1 green and 1 red pepper, coarsely
chopped

4 large tomatoes, coarsely chopped,
or 2 cups canned tomatoes

3 small zucchini or summer squash,
cut into ¼-inch slices

2 tablespoons chopped fresh basil,
or 1 teaspoon dried

½ teaspoon dried oregano

½ teaspoon dried thyme

3 tablespoons chopped fresh parsley,
or 1 tablespoon dried

½ cup whole almonds lightly
roasted

In a 4-quart pot, heat the oil, add garlic and onion, and cook until soft, about 5 minutes. Add eggplant and peppers and stir well. Cover the pot and cook over medium heat for 10 minutes, stirring occasionally.

Add the tomatoes, zucchini or summer squash, and the herbs and mix well. Cover and cook over low heat about 15 minutes, or until eggplant is tender. Stir in the almonds. Serve hot over cooked brown rice or pasta, or stuff into whole wheat pita for a luscious sandwich.

*Yield:* 5 servings

---

**Each serving provides approximately 178 calories, 5.3 g protein, .4 g saturated fat, 9 g unsaturated fat, 108 mg sodium.**

---

# Rice Ambrosia with Pineapple and Orange

This lovely dish will delight your taste buds and do your heart good. Brown rice provides fiber, magnesium, and a lot of B vitamins. Pineapple provides vitamins C and A, both valuable antioxidants, and copper, an important micronutrient that is necessary for the utilization of iron and for the rhythmic electrical activity of the heart muscle.

One 20-ounce can unsweetened
　crushed pineapple
2 cups cooked brown rice
2 oranges, peeled, sectioned, and
　pitted, or 1 can mandarin oranges
½ cup coarsely chopped walnuts

¼ cup oat bran or wheat germ
1 pound seedless grapes
1 banana, sliced
1 cup plain nonfat yogurt
¼ cup oat bran crunch or
　Grape-Nuts for garnish

Drain the pineapple and reserve the juice.

In a large glass bowl, combine the rice and reserved pineapple juice. Add the oranges, walnuts, oat bran or wheat germ, grapes, banana slices, and ½ cup of the yogurt. Spread the remaining yogurt over the top and garnish with a sprinkling of oat bran crunch or Grape-Nuts.

*Yield:* 8 servings

**Each serving provides approximately 180 calories, 5.5 g protein, 3.5 g unsaturated fat, just a trace of sodium.**

# HEARTY MAIN COURSES

The joy of eating is enhanced by these delicious dishes for main courses.

The most popular main dishes today are chicken and fish. Yesterday's utopian promise of a chicken in every pot—back when chicken, because of its succulent goodness, was everybody's favorite *special occasion* meal—is now today's reality. Because of our current concern over the danger of cholesterol-raising saturated fats, chicken and its cousins in the fowl family have won a favored spot on the menu.

*Chicken provides as much protein as red meat, but with far less fat.* And the fat in chicken is not the cholesterol-raising saturated type. Far from it! The fat in chicken is predominantly heart-healthy monounsaturated, which means that chicken skin is not the cholesterol-raising villain many people believe it to be. Chicken skin is only 17 percent fat and, when rendered, can delight you with the most delectable of flavors.

As the nineteenth-century French gastronome Jean Anthelme Brillat-Savarin wrote, "Poultry is to the cook what canvas is to the painter. It is served boiled, roasted, fried, hot or cold, whole or in pieces, with or without sauce, boned, skinned, stuffed and always with equal success."

The chicken recipes in this book come wrapped in a lovely blanket of antioxidants. Enjoy them in good health.

Yes, chicken is good, but there are more health advantages in fish. At least three fish meals every week are recommended for good cardiovascular health.

Not only will fish, prepared with these recipes as your guide, delight you with its succulent goodness, it will provide your body with all the important nutrients: protein, vitamins, minerals, vitamin trace elements, and, most important, essential fatty acids so important to your heart and, yes, to your brain. Remember how your mom told you to "eat your fish—it's a brain food"? Mom was right.

Although chicken and fish are the healthier choices, you can still enjoy the tempting flavors and succulence of beef, veal, and lamb, all of which are excellent sources of protein; the B vitamins niacin, thiamin, riboflavin, $B_6$, and $B_{12}$; as well as important minerals such as zinc, phosphorus, magnesium, copper, and selenium. Select pieces with the least fat and remove excess fat before cooking. And when buying beef, look for the USDA "extra lean" label, which indicates that there is less than 10 grams of fat, less than 4 grams of saturated fat, and less than 95 milligrams of cholesterol per serving.

# Skillet Orange Chicken

Tangerine may be substituted for the orange in this savory dish.

1 broiler-fryer chicken, cut up

2 tablespoons canola oil or chicken fat

1 tablespoon grated orange or tangerine rind

½ cup orange juice

1 orange or tangerine, or half of each, thinly sliced

2 tablespoons honey

2 tablespoons water

1½ tablespoons whole wheat or soy flour

1 small onion, chopped

In a large skillet, cook chicken in oil or chicken fat until well browned, about 15 minutes.

Add the grated orange or tangerine rind, orange juice, onion, and honey. Cover; cook over low heat 30 minutes, or until tender. Remove chicken to serving dish; keep warm.

Blend water into flour gradually; add to the sauce in the skillet. Cook, stirring constantly, until thickened. Add orange slices; serve over chicken.

*Yield:* 4 servings

---

**Each serving provides approximately 200 calories, 16 g protein, 1 g saturated fat, 4 g unsaturated fat, 39 mg sodium.**

---

# Tropical Chicken Salad

A lovely medley of fruits and nuts makes this salad a hard-working antioxidant-rich medley of delightful flavors and textures.

2 cups cooked chicken, cut in bite-size pieces
1 cup diced celery
One 20-ounce can pineapple chunks, drained, juice reserved
2 oranges, peeled and sectioned
½ cup chopped pecans, lightly roasted
1 cup seedless whole grapes
4 tablespoons reduced-calorie mayonnaise combined with 4 tablespoons of the reserved pineapple juice
Romaine lettuce leaves

Combine chicken, celery, pineapple chunks, oranges, pecans, grapes, and dressing in a glass serving bowl. Serve on Romaine lettuce leaves.

*Yield:* 6 servings

**Each portion provides 220 calories, 16 g protein, 1.2 g saturated fat, 7.2 g unsaturated fat, 93 g sodium.**

# Chicken-Apple Salad

Whether it keeps the doctor away or not, an apple every day certainly doesn't hurt. It provides plenty of fiber, some vitamin C, and is cholesterol- and sodium-free. Toss a chopped apple together with last night's chicken and a few raisins for a delicious meal.

1 cup cooked diced chicken or turkey

1 cup diced apples (about 2 medium)

⅓ cup chopped celery

¼ cup raisins

1 tablespoons lemon juice

¼ cup mayonnaise

Salad greens

Combine chicken or turkey, apples, celery, and raisins in a bowl. Make a dressing with lemon juice and mayonnaise; add to other ingredients and mix well. Chill thoroughly. Serve on a bed of salad greens.

*Yield:* 4 servings

**Each serving provides approximately 186 calories, 12 g protein, 2 g saturated fat, 6 g unsaturated fat, 364 mg sodium.**

# Chopped Chicken Liver Salad or Sandwich

Liver, like all organ meats, is a wonderful source of selenium. Selenium's broadest role, according to some medical experts, may lie in protecting cells from the low-level but constant barrage of carcinogens hidden in air, food, and water.

8 chicken livers

½ onion

2 hard-boiled eggs

⅓ cup toasted soy nuts

3 crisp romaine leaves

Salt-Free Herbal Seasoning (page 143) and freshly ground pepper to taste

Wash and broil the livers until they are brown all the way through.

Combine all the ingredients with the broiled livers in a food chopper or processor, or as I do, in a wooden bowl and chop with a hockmesser (chopping cleaver). Season to taste.

Serve with grated white radish or on crackers, stuffed into celery or on slices of turnip for more cancer protection, or on Jewish seeded rye bread, for a more traditional flavor.

*Yield:* 6 servings

---

**Each serving provides 95 calories, 16 g protein, .5 g saturated fat, 1.1 g unsaturated fat, 33 mg sodium.**

---

# Waldorf Chicken Salad

Created at New York's Waldorf-Astoria hotel, this is a variation on the classic. Tart apples and sweet grapes tossed in a tofu mayonnaise with raisins and walnuts and spiced with nutmeg, my version is power packed.

2 cups bite-size pieces of cooked chicken

1 large Granny Smith apple, unpeeled and coarsely chopped

2 stalks celery, sliced diagonally

1 small green or red pepper, diced

½ small onion, diced

1 cup halved seedless red or green grapes

½ cup coarsely chopped walnuts

1 cup raisins

⅔ cup orange juice

½ cup soft tofu or plain yogurt

⅛ teaspoon ground nutmeg (optional)

Dark green lettuce leaves

In a glass bowl, combine chicken, apple, celery, pepper, onion, grapes, and half the walnuts. In a small bowl, beat the orange juice, yogurt or tofu, and nutmeg with a fork until well blended. Pour over the chicken mixture and mix thoroughly. Garnish with remaining walnuts. Serve on lettuce leaves.

*Yield:* 4 servings

Each portion provides 330 calories, 28 g protein, 1 g saturated fat, 11.5 g unsaturated fat, 83 g sodium.

# Raspberry-Cayenne Chicken

This recipe is an adaptation of one of my favorites from Chicken Cookery published by Delmarva Poultry Association, Delaware, 1994. The raspberry sauce elevates this chicken dish to the realm of the heavenly. With that intense flavor comes potassium, vitamin C, fiber, and protease inhibitors to help snuff out cancer before it begins. Cayenne pepper gives it just the right heat.

2 chicken legs (thigh and drumstick attached)
½ cup red raspberry jam
2 tablespoons balsamic vinegar
1 tablespoon reduced sodium soy sauce
¼ teaspoon cayenne pepper, or to taste
Parsley

Bake the chicken in a 375°F oven for about 45 minutes or until brown.
Mix together the jam, vinegar, soy sauce, and cayenne pepper. Spoon the sauce over

the chicken and bake about 15 minutes longer, or until chicken is fork tender and beautifully glazed.

Arrange chicken on your best platter and garnish with sprigs of parsley.

*Yield:* 2 to 4 servings

---

**Each serving for 2 provides 300 calories, 25 g protein, 2.18 g saturated fat, 4.36 g unsaturated fat, 368 mg sodium.**

---

# Grilled Chicken Livers with Mushrooms

A tender, crunchy delight, this dish beats hot dogs both in flavor and nutrient value. Serve them at your next picnic.

| | |
|---|---|
| 1 pound chicken livers | ¼ teaspoon onion powder |
| 1 tablespoon chicken fat or olive oil | ¼ teaspoon dried oregano |
| ¼ cup dry white wine | 8 medium-size mushrooms, halved, |
| ½ cup crushed oat bran crunch or | or 16 small mushrooms |
| your favorite high-fiber dry cereal | 8 cherry tomatoes |

Cut the chicken livers in halves. Combine 1 tablespoon chicken fat or oil and wine in a medium-size bowl and add the chicken livers. Marinate for 30 minutes, refrigerated.

On wax paper, combine cereal crumbs, onion powder, and oregano. Drain the chicken livers, reserving the marinade, and roll in crumb mixture.

Thread livers, mushrooms, and tomatoes alternately on 4 skewers. Brush with reserved marinade.

Grill 15 minutes, turning once or until liver is slightly browned.

*Yield:* 4 servings

Each serving provides 191 calories, 24 g protein, 2 g saturated fat, 3 g unsaturated fat, 402 mg cholesterol, 82 mg sodium.

# Turkey and Avocado–Filled Pitas

Pitas are the perfect take-away foods; you can stuff them with all manner of foods flavorful and healthy. This particular filling combines creamy avocados, tangy radishes, and good greens with turkey—a delicious, nutritious combination.

1½ cups chopped radishes
1¼ cups diced avocado
¼ cup prepared salad dressing
Four 6-inch pita breads, cut
  crosswise in halves

½ pound sliced turkey or chicken
1 cup shredded romaine
1 cup spinach leaves

In a small bowl, combine radishes, avocado, and dressing; set aside.

Fill pita halves with turkey, shredded romaine, spinach, and reserved radish-avocado mixture, dividing evenly. Serve immediately or wrap individually in plastic wrap or place in sandwich bags and send them to school or to work with a hearty lunch, or refrigerate for as long as 5 hours.

*Yield:* 8 servings

Each serving provides approximately 130 calories, 6 g protein, 5 g unsaturated fat, 9 mg sodium.

# Fish Steaks with Onion and Orange

A delicious dinner reinforced with antioxidant- and phytochemical-rich onion, orange peel, and red pepper. Use any firm-fleshed fish: salmon, cod, halibut, tile, or mako shark.

1 large onion, halved lengthwise and cut into thin wedges
2 strips (½ by 2 inches) orange zest
½ sweet red pepper
1 tablespoon olive oil
Freshly ground pepper to taste
Vegetable seasoning to taste
1 teaspoon thyme leaves, or a dash of dried thyme
4 fish steaks, about ¾ inch thick (salmon, cod, halibut, tile, mako shark)
Fresh thyme or parsley sprigs for garnish

Preheat oven to 400°F.

Combine the onion, orange zest, sweet red pepper, olive oil, and about half the seasonings in 13-by-9-inch baking dish.

Bake until edges of vegetables just begin to brown, stirring once or twice, for about 20 minutes.

Remove dish from oven. Increase oven temperature to 450°F. Sprinkle fish with remaining seasoning. Push the precooked onion mixture to one side and arrange steaks in same dish, spooning some onion mixture over each fish steak. Bake until fish is opaque in center when you test with tip of knife, about 10 minutes.

*Yield:* 4 servings

---

**When made with salmon each serving provides approximately 226 calories, 22 g protein, .3 g unsaturated fat, 2 mg sodium.**

---

# Salmon Salad with Gingery Raisin Sauce

Enjoy it hot or cold and enjoy it often to reap the benefits of the broad anticancer power generously provided by the dark green leafy vegetables and the carrots. And count the blessings in the omega-3 fatty acids the salmon is graciously providing to cut the odds of a heart attack, clogged arteries, rheumatoid arthritis, and other afflictions you can live very nicely without.

1 tablespoon arrowroot powder
1 cup orange juice
½ cup raisins
2 tablespoons sliced green onions
2 teaspoons Dijon mustard
1 teaspoon grated fresh ginger root
    or ⅓ teaspoon powdered ginger

1 teaspoon chopped fresh dill
    weed
¼ teaspoon Salt-Free Herbal
    Seasoning (page 143)
4 salmon steaks (about 1½ pounds)
Salad greens for 4

Preheat broiler.

In a medium-size saucepan, combine the arrowroot with 2 tablespoons of the orange juice. Add the remaining orange juice and bring to a boil, stirring until thickened. Stir in the raisins, onions, mustard, ginger root, dill, and herbal seasoning. Mix well and set aside.

Place the fish in a buttered baking dish. Place the oven rack about 6 inches below the source of heat. Broil for 5 to 8 minutes on each side. To test for doneness, see if you can remove the center bone without taking any of the flesh with it

Place each steak on top of a bowl of salad greens and shredded carrots. Drizzle with the raisin dressing.

*Yield:* 4 servings

Each serving provides 262 calories, 20 g protein, 4.4 g saturated fat, 5.2 g unsaturated fat, 53 mg sodium, 66 mg cholesterol.

# Tuna-Apple Salad

This is a lovely substantial dish for a company lunch. Tuna is a good source of selenium, a trace mineral that helps detoxify free radicals. Selenium is best gotten through food rather than through supplements.

One 6½-ounce can water-packed
   tuna, drained
4 tablespoons chopped celery
1 large carrot, grated
1 large apple, washed, cored, and
   chunked

½ cup mashed tofu
2 teaspoons lemon juice
2 tablespoons mayonnaise
1 tablespoon pickle relish, or to
   taste
Romaine lettuce leaves for garnish

In a medium to large bowl combine the tuna, celery, carrot, and apple. Mix well. In a small bowl, combine the tofu, lemon juice, mayonnaise, and relish. Add to the tuna. Mix thoroughly. Serve on romaine leaves.

**Yield:** Six ¹/₂-cup servings

---

**Each serving provides 93 calories, 6 g protein, .5 g saturated fat, 1.2 g unsaturated fat, 54 mg sodium.**

---

# Tuna Slaw Lunch

The selenium in the tuna helps build your defense against cancer. The indoles provided by the cabbage deliver a knock-out blow to enemy agents that cause cancer.

One 6½-ounce can water-packed
   tuna
½ cup plain low-fat yogurt
1 tablespoon reduced-fat
   mayonnaise
1 tablespoon red wine or rice vinegar
1 tablespoon honey

½ pimiento, chopped
1 tablespoon chopped green pepper
1 tablespoon chopped green onion
½ teaspoon dry mustard
Freshly ground pepper to taste
2 cups shredded cabbage

In a medium-size bowl, combine all the ingredients except the cabbage. Toss with cabbage and chill.

*Yield:* 4 servings

---

**Each serving provides approximately 119 calories, 15.4 g protein, insignificant amount of fat, 85 mg sodium.**

---

# Fish, Mushroom, and Rice Pie

Brown rice makes a delicious crunchy crust for this tasty satisfying one-dish meal.

## Crust

1 tablespoon finely minced onion
2 cups cooked brown rice
2 tablespoons olive or peanut oil
½ teaspoon dried thyme, or 1 tablespoon fresh
1 egg, beaten

## Filling

¾ pound cooked fish, flaked (or one 7-ounce can of tuna or salmon)

3 eggs, beaten

1 cup milk

1 cup sliced mushrooms

1 tablespoon finely minced onion

1 tablespoon olive or peanut oil

Dash of freshly ground pepper

### TO MAKE THE CRUST

Combine all ingredients and press into bottom and sides of an oiled 8- or 9-inch pie plate.

### TO MAKE THE FILLING

Preheat oven to 350°F.

Spread flaked fish over the rice shell. Combine eggs and milk in a small bowl.

Sauté mushrooms and onion until golden in the oil and sprinkle pepper over all. Add to egg and milk and mix well. Pour over the fish. Bake for 50 to 55 minutes. Serve hot.

*Yield:* 8 servings

**Each serving provides 164 calories, 14.5 g protein, 9.5 g saturated fat, 8.5 g unsaturated fat, 43.5 mg sodium.**

# Curried Flounder with Sweet Potatoes, Bananas, and Coconut

Perfect for company or special family dinner, this unique dish implies a wish for good health and a long sweet life.

2 cups orange juice

½ teaspoon ground cinnamon

¼ teaspoon ground ginger

1 teaspoon curry powder, or to taste

¼ cup raisins

4 medium-size sweet potatoes, unpeeled, scrubbed, and cut into ½-inch slices

2 pounds flounder or sole fillets

1 large banana, peeled, sliced, and dipped in acidulated water (see Note)

½ cup grated unsweetened coconut or toasted sunflower seeds

In a large heavy pot, bring the orange juice to a boil. Add cinnamon, ginger, curry powder, raisins, and sweet potatoes. Reduce heat to simmer, cover, and cook until potatoes are barely fork-tender, about 15 minutes. Push potatoes aside and add the fish fillets. The fish should be covered by the juice. Cover and simmer until fish flakes, about 8 to 10 minutes. Remove fish and potatoes to a heated platter. Spoon some liquid over all. Garnish with banana and sprinkle with coconut or toasted sunflower seeds. Serve the remaining juice on the side.

**Note:** To make acidulated water, mix 1 tablespoon lemon juice or white vinegar with 1 quart water.

**Yield:** 6 servings

---

**Each serving provides 338 calories, 20.7 g protein, 4.48 g saturated fat, .6 g unsaturated fat, 82.75 mg sodium, 65 mg cholesterol.**

# Beautiful Baked Fish Fillets with Avocado

Good for the body, great for the soul! Fish is an excellent source of omega-3 fatty acids, which may help unclog the arteries; lower levels of LDL, the bad cholesterol; and may also have a positive effect on inflammatory disease, such as rheumatoid arthritis, asthma, and scleroderma. Fish also provides selenium, the anticancer mineral. With yogurt and avocado and their health-enhancing ability, this triple-threat alliance makes an elegant dish.

| | |
|---|---|
| 1 pound fish fillets (flounder, sole, etc.) | 1 tablespoon chopped parsley |
| 1 cup plain yogurt | 1 tablespoon lemon juice |
| 2 tablespoons finely chopped onion | ¼ teaspoon dry mustard |
| 2 tablespoons finely chopped green or red pepper | Paprika |
| | Lemon slices |
| 2 tablespoons chopped dill pickle | 1 ripe avocado, pitted, peeled, and sliced |

Preheat oven to 375°F.

Arrange fish in a baking dish. In a small mixing bowl, combine yogurt, onion, pepper, pickle, parsley, lemon juice, and mustard. Spread the yogurt mixture over the fish. Sprinkle with paprika. Bake for about 15 minutes, or until fish flakes easily. Garnish with lemon and avocado slices.

*Yield:* 4 servings

Each serving provides 192 calories, 23.9 g protein, 3.6 g saturated fat, 9.9 g unsaturated fat, 89 mg sodium, 45 mg cholesterol.

# Avocado Stuffed with Tuna and Walnuts

Velvety avocado and crunchy nuts make this dish a gourmet sensation. Avocados are a marvelous source of the fats that lower harmful cholesterol. They also provide vitamin A, a hard-working antioxidant, which puts a nice glow on your complexion while protecting you from a multitude of infections. Though this is a high-calorie delight, every calorie is hard working.

| | |
|---|---|
| 2 ripe avocados | 1 cup drained yogurt |
| 1 cup chopped walnuts | 3 tablespoons catsup or cocktail sauce |
| One 6½-ounce can solid white tuna, drained, or 1 cup flaked cooked fish | Salt-Free Herbal Seasoning (page 143) and pepper to taste |
| | Lemon wedges |

Halve and pit avocados and scoop out the flesh. Be careful not to break the skin. Dice the avocado flesh into ½-inch cubes. In a bowl, combine the tuna or flaked fish with the avocado. Gently blend in ⅔ cup of the walnuts.

In another bowl, combine the drained yogurt with the catsup or cocktail sauce.

Combine the two mixtures and season to taste. Lightly rub the insides of the reserved avocado shells with a wedge of lemon.

Divide the salad among the avocado shells and garnish with the remaining walnuts. Serve with lemon wedges.

*Yield:* 4 servings

---

**Each serving provides 500 calories, 20 g protein, 11.3 g saturated fat, 36 g unsaturated fat, 34 mg sodium.**

---

# Tuna-Stuffed Potatoes

A great way to entice children to eat fish. Serve it in a potato with a salad and you have a great dinner. These are also ideal take-alongs for picnics.

One 6½-ounce can white albacore
    tuna in water
2 large potatoes
1 cup sliced green onions
1 cup shredded zucchini
2 tablespoons water or vegetable
    broth

1 clove garlic, pressed
1 teaspoon vegetable seasoning
2 tablespoons grated Parmesan
    cheese
½ teaspoon dried thyme
½ cup milk

Drain the tuna and set aside. Bake the potatoes in a 400°F oven for 1 hour or microwave for about 10 minutes on high. Set aside to cool.

In a skillet, simmer the onions and zucchini in the water or broth until soft. Remove from heat and stir in the vegetable seasoning, Parmesan, and thyme.

Slice the tops off the potatoes lengthwise. Scoop out the flesh, being careful not to split the skin. In mixer, beat the potatoes with milk until fluffy. Add tuna and vegetable mixture. Combine ingredients well. Spoon into potato skins. (If mounds get too high, reserve the extra for a side dish for another meal.) Heat the stuffed potatoes in the preheated oven for about 20 minutes, or in the microwave oven for 2 or 3 minutes on high, until heated through.

*Yield:* 2 bountiful servings

Each serving provides approximately 360 calories, 37 g protein, 2.8 g saturated fat, 1 g unsaturated fat, 118 mg sodium.

# Veal and Grapefruit with Snow Peas

The grapefruit lends an indescribable zest as well as several cancer-deterring nutrients to this dish.

1 teaspoon honey

¼ cup dry sherry

2 garlic cloves, crushed

¾ pound veal cutlets, cut into 2-inch pieces

1 teaspoon arrowroot powder

1 tablespoon Worcestershire sauce

1 tablespoon unsweetened grapefruit juice

1 large grapefruit, cut into segments

2 teaspoons canola or olive oil

½ cucumber cut into matchstick strips

In a small bowl, combine honey, sherry, and garlic.

Marinate the veal in the sherry mixture for about 10 minutes. Remove from marinade, reserving liquid. Sprinkle the arrowroot over the veal and set aside.

Mix grapefruit juice and Worcestershire sauce and add to marinade.

Cut the grapefruit into segments, adding any escaping juice to the marinade. Set aside.

Heat 1 teaspoon oil in a wok. When wok is good and hot, add half the veal. Stir-fry for 30 seconds. Add remaining veal and stir-fry for 3 minutes.

Remove veal from wok. Add remaining oil and marinade to wok. When the sauce is bubbling, return the veal to the pan. Stir-fry for 1 minute. Add the cucumbers and reserved grapefruit segments. Serve over brown rice.

*Yield:* 2 servings

---

**Each serving provides approximately 420 calories, 41g protein, 14 g saturated fat, 3 g unsaturated fat, 247 mg sodium.**

---

# Apple-Lamb Curry

Apples in this main dish contribute a delightful contrast in flavor and texture and make a little meat go a long way.

| | |
|---|---|
| 1 pound boneless stewing lamb | 1 cup diced apples (about 2 |
| ½ cup chopped onion | medium), preferably tart |
| 1 teaspoon Tamari reduced-sodium | ¼ cup raisins |
| soy sauce | 2 tablespoons arrowroot powder |
| 1 teaspoon curry powder | or flour |
| 1 teaspoon honey | 2 cups cooked brown rice |
| 1 to 1¼ cups water | |

Trim excess fat from the meat and cut into one-inch cubes. Brown in a heavy saucepan. Drain off any fat. Add onion, soy sauce, curry powder, honey, and 1 cup water. Cover and simmer for 1 hour, or until meat is tender. Add apples and raisins and cook about 15 minutes longer. If mixture is not thick enough, mix arrowroot with ¼ cup water and stir into juices. Cook, stirring constantly, until thickened. Serve over hot brown rice.

*Yield:* 6 servings

---

**Each serving provides approximately 240 calories, 23 g protein, 7.5 g saturated fat, .5 g unsaturated fat, 53 mg sodium.**

---

# Tofu and Ground Beef

This dish brings you the flavor of meat with half the calories and fat, not to mention the cancer-blocking protease inhibitors in the tofu. Made with only half a pound of ground beef, it is a low-fat, mineral-rich, high-protein dish.

½ pound lean ground beef

1 clove garlic, minced

2 tablespoons finely chopped
   scallions or onion

2 cups sliced fresh mushrooms

3 cups ½-inch cubes tofu

2 tablespoons reduced-sodium
   Tamari soy sauce

1 teaspoon honey

1 tablespoon arrowroot powder

½ cup water or stock

In a nonstick skillet, cook the beef, garlic, scallions or onion, and mushrooms until the meat changes color. Drain off any fat. Add the tofu, Tamari, and honey. Cover and cook slowly for 10 minutes. Stir the arrowroot into the water or stock; add to the tofu-and-meat mixture. Cook over low heat until the mixture thickens.

*Yield:* 6 servings

**Each serving provides 90 calories, 10.5 g protein, 3.5 g saturated fat, 381 mg sodium.**

# Dressings, Dips, Spreads, and Vinaigrettes

These recipes will bring you expertise with embellishments that will give your meals something extra—the extra that takes them out of the ordinary into elegant. And because, with guidance provided by these recipes, you can make them yourself, you will save a bundle.

Provide your family, friends, and guests with a choice of salad dressings, like Raspberry Vinaigrette or Honey-Caraway Dressing, made with heart-healthy olive oil and antioxidant-rich orange rind. The Garlic Croutons will turn any green salad into a sublime dish.

Prepare a lovely spread, sweet as jam but made without sugar, from orange juice and dried grapes, or raisins. Dried grape skin is prescribed by physicians and available in health food stores and some pharmacies as a very versatile antioxidant.

Live it up and enjoy!

# Honey-Caraway Dressing

This zippy dressing helps you boost your intake of cancer fighters. The soy sauce provides wonder-working genistein and the caraway seeds provide protease inhibitors, which tend to deliver a knock-out punch to incipient malignant cells.

½ teaspoon dry mustard

2 teaspoons reduced-sodium soy
   sauce

2 tablespoons lemon juice

⅛ teaspoon freshly ground pepper

1 tablespoon olive oil

2 teaspoons grated onion

2 tablespoons honey

1 teaspoon grated orange rind

½ teaspoon caraway seeds, crushed

Combine all ingredients in a screw-top jar. Shake well.

*Yield:* 6 tablespoons

Each tablespoon provides 43 calories, trace protein, trace saturated fat, 2 g unsaturated fat, 360 mg sodium.

# Yogurt Salad Dressing

The perfect dressing for spinach and its cousins in the greens family.

1 cup nonfat yogurt

1 teaspoon lemon juice

½ teaspoon finely minced chives

½ teaspoon paprika

½ teaspoon dry mustard

Combine all ingredients and mix well. Chill.

*Yield:* 1 cup; eight 2-tablespoons servings

---

**Each serving provides 15 calories, 1 g protein, insignificant fat, 6 mg sodium.**

---

# Raspberry-Yogurt Dip

This dip is lovely to look at, delightful to eat, and a very good inducement to eat more salad.

  1 cup nonfat yogurt
  1 cup raspberries, fresh or frozen
  1 teaspoon grated orange rind

Drain the yogurt in a cheesecloth-lined strainer for about 10 minutes.

Puree the raspberries in a food processor and fold into the drained yogurt. Stir in the orange rind.

*Yield:* 1 cup; eight 2-tablespoon servings

---

**Each serving provides approximately 21 calories, 1.4 g protein, a trace of fat, 19 mg sodium.**

---

# Tuna-Yogurt Dip

Tuna, like all fish, is a wonderful source of life-saving omega-3 fatty acids.

| | |
|---|---|
| 1 small onion, chopped | 2 tablespoons whole wheat or soy |
| 1 tablespoon olive or vegetable oil | flour |
| 1 cup sliced mushrooms | 1 cup nonfat yogurt |
| Freshly ground pepper to taste | One 6½-ounce can water-packed tuna |

Sauté onion in oil until translucent. Add mushrooms and ground pepper to taste and cook, covered, for about a minute. Add the flour and continue to cook for another minute. Add ½ cup yogurt and mix well.

Combine this mixture with the drained tuna in a blender or food processor, and process until smooth. Return to skillet and add the other ½ cup of yogurt and heat. Serve it hot as a main dish on top of brown rice or crisp whole grain toast. Serve it cold with vegetables as a dip.

**Yield:** 3 cups, 6 servings

---

Each serving provides approximately 100 calories, 11.5 g protein, .4 g saturated fat, 2 g unsaturated fat, 16 mg sodium.

---

# Orange-Raisin Spread

A delightfully flavorful no-fat and no-sugar spread for toast or bagels. I love to spread it on a peanut butter sandwich. Raisins, which are dried grapes, are powerful antioxidants shown to reduce the growth of cancer.

¾ cup orange or any citrus juice

1½ cups raisins

Pinch of cinnamon

Pinch of ground cloves

In a saucepan, combine all ingredients. Simmer, uncovered, for 10 minutes. Whiz in a blender or food processor until smooth. Refrigerate.

*Yield:* 1¼ cups, or 20 tablespoons

**Each tablespoon provides approximately 4.5 calories, .5 g protein, no fat, .5 mg sodium.**

# Fruit-and-Seed Spread

Terrific on toast and muffins, this crumbly spread is enriched with antioxidant vitamin C in the apple and lemon, cancer inhibitor genistein from the tofu, vitamin E from the sunflower and sesame seeds, and the valuable antioxidant provided by the grated orange rind.

1 medium Golden Delicious apple,
  peeled and seeded

1 tablespoon lemon juice

3 tablespoons soft tofu

1 teaspoon honey

½ cup toasted sunflower seeds

½ cup toasted sesame seeds

½ teaspoon cinnamon

1 tablespoon grated orange rind

Pinch of nutmeg

Cut apple into slices and combine it with remaining ingredients in a blender or food processor. Whiz until all ingredients are well combined and the mixture has a smooth consistency.

*Yield:* About 1 cup, or 16 tablespoons

**Each tablespoon provides 50 calories, 3.4 g protein, 2 g unsaturated fat.**

# Raspberry Vinaigrette

To get your vegetable scorners to eat more salad, and to make your salad absolutely irresistible, douse it with this sensational raspberry vinaigrette.

   3 tablespoons olive oil
   3 tablespoons red wine vinegar
   3 tablespoons fruit-juice sweetened raspberry spread
      (Sorrell Ridge is a good brand)
   2 cloves garlic, minced

Combine all ingredients in a salad cruet or mason jar and shake.

*Yield:* About 8 ounces

**Each ounce (2 tablespoons) provides approximately 51 calories, .6 g protein, 4.5 g unsaturated fat.**

# Garlic Croutons

Dress up a salad by adding these garlicky, low-sodium croutons for extra flavor and a satisfying crunch.

> 2 tablespoons butter
> 2 cloves crushed garlic
> 2 cups bread cubes, made from stale bread, preferably whole wheat
> 4 tablespoons grated Parmesan cheese (optional)
> 1 teaspoon Salt-Free Herbal Seasoning (see below)

Preheat oven to 350°F.

Melt butter in skillet. Add crushed garlic. Toss bread cubes, melted butter, and Parmesan cheese until cubes are evenly coated. Spread on baking sheet and toast in the oven for about 15 minutes. Sprinkle with herbal seasoning.

*Yield:* 2 cups croutons; 4 servings

---

**Each $1/4$ cup provides approximately 146 calories, 2.1 g protein, 3 g saturated fat, 2.5 g unsaturated fat, 6 mg sodium.**

---

# Salt-Free Herbal Seasoning

This blend will help you cut down on salt and savor the flavor.

> 3 teaspoons onion power
> 3 teaspoons garlic powder
> 3 teaspoons dried minced parsley

1 teaspoon dried thyme

1 teaspoon dried marjoram

1 teaspoon freshly ground pepper

In a container with a tight-fitting lid, combine all ingredients. Mix and seal tightly. Store in a cool dry place. Shake well before using.

*Yield:* ¹/₂ cup

# DESSERTS

Rarely do children ask, "What's for dinner?" They always want to know, "What's for dessert, Mom?"

But let's face it. A meal with a great dessert has a very happy ending.

The good news is, you can serve gorgeous desserts that are actually good for you, that contain no negative ingredients, that actually contribute vitamins and minerals, many of them life-saving antioxidants.

I recommend that you don't use white flour; use whole wheat flour, which includes wheat germ and bran. And soy flour is included so that you get the benefit of the protease inhibitors, which do valiant guard duty as they protect you from all kinds of viruses.

Many fruits—fresh, frozen, and dried—are presented in lovely, tempting dishes. Learn all about them in the following recipes. They will titillate your desire for dessert.

Keep the desire for dessert happily alive during dinner. But please don't eat it first!

# Stewed Dried Fruit

A lovely, light dessert; a perfect ending to a hearty meal.

  1 cup dried apricots
  1 cup pitted prunes
  1 cup raisins
  1 tablespoon grated orange zest
  3 slices of lemon
  ½ cup warm water or sugar-free fruit juice

Place all ingredients in a microsafe bowl. Add the warm water or sugar-free fruit juice. Microwave partly covered, on medium for 3 or 4 minutes, or until the ingredients are soft.

*Yield:* 4 servings

---

Each serving provides 285 calories, .5 g unsaturated fat.

---

# Dried Fruit Nuggets

It is said that King David accepted sun-dried grapes, or raisins, in payment of taxes. Why not? Dried fruits are a good source of protein and vitamin A, an important antioxidant cancer inhibitor. Many fruits also provide important minerals, including potassium, magnesium, iron, and calcium.

What's more, there is no cooking involved in the preparation of these naturally sweet confections.

½ cup pitted dates or date nuggets

¼ cup pitted prunes

1 cup raisins

1 cup dried apricots

1 cup figs

1 to 2 tablespoons honey

½ cup sunflower seeds

1 cup natural peanut butter

## Toppings

Sesame seeds, chopped nuts, or unsweetened shredded coconut

Grind the dried fruit in a food grinder or food processor. Add remaining ingredients except the toppings. Mix well, then form into small balls and roll in your choice of the toppings.

*Yield:* 36 confections

---

**Each confection provides approximately 119 calories, 2.9 g protein, a trace of saturated fat, 4 g unsaturated fat, 9 mg sodium.**

---

# Becca's Apple-Blueberry Crisp

A rhapsody in blue and white with a crunchy top hat, this summer favorite is loaded with antioxidants. This crisp is best served hot with a scoop of ice cream but is also delicious as a cool midnight snack.

3 apples, thinly sliced
1 cup blueberries
1 tablespoon lemon juice
1 cup rolled oats
2 tablespoons whole wheat pastry
    flour
¼ cup soy flour

¼ cup raisins
1 teaspoon cinnamon
1 teaspoon grated orange rind
¼ cup apple juice
3 tablespoons honey
1 tablespoon canola oil

Preheat oven to 350°F.

Spritz a 9-by-13-inch baking dish with nonstick cooking spray. Add the apples, blueberries, and lemon juice, and mix well. In a large bowl, combine the oats, flours, raisins, cinnamon, orange rind, apple juice, honey, and oil. Spread this mixture over the fruit.

Bake for 30 minutes, or until the apples are tender.

**Yield:** About 10 servings

**Each serving provides approximately 107 calories, .6 g protein, a trace of fat, 17 mg sodium.**

# Blueberry Pudding

A very versatile dessert that doubles as a delicious low-calorie spread for your breakfast toast. Use whatever berries are in season.

    2 cups low-fat small curd cottage cheese
    2 cups blueberries
    1 cup plain nonfat yogurt
    3 tablespoons lemon juice
    2 tablespoons honey

Blend all ingredients in food processor until smooth, about 4 minutes. Place the mixture in a pretty serving bowl or divide among 6 sherbet glasses.

*Yield:* 6 servings

---

**Each serving provides approximately 112 calories, 10 g protein, an insignificant amount of fat, 96 mg sodium.**

---

## FROM KUMQUAT TO GRAPEFRUIT

All citrus is loaded with vitamin C, one of nature's most therapeutic gifts, known for its ability to neutralize free radicals, those destructive cancer-causing molecules formed by normal metabolism, infections, cigarette smoking, and pollution.

Studies reveal that vitamin C may help protect against cancers of the larynx, throat, esophagus, pancreas, stomach, rectum, breast, cervix, and lung.

All citrus are alike in that they are all empowered with vitamin C. And yet, each is different in the kind of protection it provides. Each, from a different member of the citrus family, provides its own special arsenal.

There are in citrus at least six different flavonoids that have been found in the laboratory to squelch an invading carcinogen in its tracks.

# Lime and Avocado Parfait

Soft, velvety avocado teams up with tangy lime to make a sensational dessert or a refreshing bell ringer to start your meal. Lime, like lemon, is rich in vitamin C, a valuable ally in the fight against cancer. Avocado's fatty acids are a boon to your cardiovascular system.

> 2 large ripe avocados, peeled and seeded
> 4 limes
> ⅓ cup honey
> 2 eggs, separated
> Pinch of cream of tartar

If there is a current danger of salmonella, coddle the eggs (cook for 1 minute in 120°F water).

In a blender or food processor, or with a fork, puree the flesh of the avocados. Add the strained juice of 3 of the limes, the honey, and egg yolks.

Beat the egg whites with the cream of tartar to the stiff peak stage. Fold into the avocado-lime mixture.

Divide the mixture among 4 parfait glasses and chill for about 2 hours.

Garnish with the remaining lime cut in very thin slices.

*Yield:* 4 servings

Each serving provides approximately 317 calories, 4 g protein, 5 g saturated fat, 21 g unsaturated fat, 44 mg sodium.

---

## YOGURT CHEESE ICING

You're making delicious cakes using much less fat and sugar. Must you forego the icing? Absolutely not. Use simple-to-make yogurt cheese.

Use fruit juice sweetened gelatin-free yogurt. I use Stonybrook, which is available in cappuccino, apricot-mango, and other fruity flavors. My favorite for plain cakes is apricot-mango. For chocolate cakes, I like the cappuccino.

Drain 1 pint of yogurt overnight in a colander lined with several layers of cheesecloth and placed in the refrigerator.

In the morning you will have 6 ounces of flavored yogurt cream cheese. The liquid that has drained into the bowl is whey, which can be used as a substitute for buttermilk in muffin recipes or as a delicious beverage, rich in immune-strengthening acidophilus.

To the cream cheese portion, add 2 tablespoons powdered milk or potato starch. Mix well to blend.

You now have a lovely icing for your cake. Spread it on.

---

# Pumpkin-Cheese Roll

This spicy cake wrapped around a cream cheese filling tastes like it has a zillion calories, but it is actually a weight-watcher's delight.

The pumpkin, like all orange vegetables, may help you avoid alterations in your cells that lead to cancer. The soy flour also may lower your cancer risk. The Brazil nuts are rich in selenium.

## Batter

3 eggs

¾ cup pumpkin, cooked and mashed, or canned

⅓ cup honey

1 teaspoon lemon juice

½ cup whole wheat pastry flour

¼ cup soy flour

1 teaspoon baking powder

2 teaspoons cinnamon

1 teaspoon ground ginger

½ teaspoon ground or freshly grated nutmeg

1 cup finely chopped Brazil nuts

## Filling

6 ounces light cream cheese

2 tablespoons honey

½ teaspoon vanilla extract

½ teaspoon lemon juice

Chopped Brazil nuts (optional)

### TO MAKE THE BATTER

Preheat the oven to 350°F.

Beat the eggs at high speed for 5 minutes. Beat in the pumpkin, honey, and lemon juice. Combine the dry ingredients and spices, and fold into the pumpkin mixture.

Spread the batter on a greased or parchment-lined cookie sheet. Top with slivered Brazil nuts.

Bake for 15 minutes. Roll up with the parchment paper or, if you didn't use paper, turn onto a dish towel sprinkled with a little whole wheat flour or dry powdered milk. Roll up and allow to cool.

### TO MAKE THE FILLING

Combine all the filling ingredients in blender or food processor. When the roll is cool, unroll it and spread with the filling. Roll up again, enclosing the filling. At this point, you can serve it or refrigerate or freeze it. Remove from the freezer about 30 minutes before serving.

*Yield:* 10 servings

---

**Each serving provides 208 calories, 4.7 g protein, 1.7 g saturated fat, 5.2 g unsaturated fat, 1.6 mg sodium.**

---

# Ambrosia Rice Pudding

Use this delicious combination of rice and fruits as a refreshing dessert or side dish. It's a wonderful take-along dish for summer picnics or potluck suppers.

| | |
|---|---|
| 1½ cups cooked brown rice | 2 sliced bananas |
| One 20-ounce can pineapple chunks | 1 cup blueberries or strawberries |
| 2 oranges, peeled and segmented | 2 peaches, sliced |
| ½ cup shredded unsweetened coconut | |

In a pretty glass bowl, combine the rice with the pineapple chunks and juice. Add the remaining ingredients, reserving a few blueberries or strawberries. Garnish with a sprinkling of coconut and the reserved blueberries or strawberries.

*Yield:* 10 servings

---

**Each serving provides 126 calories, 2 g protein, 1.4 g unsaturated fat, 4.5 mg sodium.**

---

# Custardy Apple Kugel

A delicious kugel you can enjoy and stay healthy. The pectin in the apple tends to lower harmful cholesterol. Pectin may also help put the brakes on runaway appetites, making it easier to stay slim.

| | |
|---|---|
| 8 ounces medium noodles, preferably artichoke | ¼ cup wheat germ |
| ⅔ cup low-fat milk plus 2 teaspoons dry milk powder | ½ teaspoon vanilla extract |
| | Juice of ½ lemon |
| 1 cup plain yogurt | ½ cup raisins |
| 8 ounces low-fat cottage cheese | 4 eggs |
| 1 large unpeeled apple, grated | 2 tablespoons unsalted butter |
| 2 tablespoons honey or pure maple syrup | 1 scant teaspoon cinnamon, or to taste |
| | 3 tablespoons chopped walnuts |

Cook the noodles according to package directions and drain. (Try artichoke noodles if you can find them. They're low in calories and high in nutrients.) In a bowl, combine the milk, milk powder, and yogurt. Add the cottage cheese and mix well. Add the grated apple, honey or maple syrup, wheat germ, vanilla, lemon juice, and raisins. Fold into the noodles.

Preheat the oven to 325°F.

Beat the eggs well and reserve. Heat an 8-by-10-inch baking dish in the oven for 10 minutes. Melt the butter in the heated dish. Pour in the cheese-noodle mixture. Pour the beaten eggs on top. Sprinkle with cinnamon and the chopped walnuts. Bake for 1 hour or until nicely browned.

*Yield:* 8 servings

---

**Each serving provides approximately 146 calories, 8 g protein, 2.6 g saturated fat, 3.4 g unsaturated fat, 60 mg sodium.**

---

# Apricot-Almond Soufflé

A soufflé is another version of the fluffy omelet except that it's made with a sauce containing the egg yolks and is baked in a deep dish that permits it to rise to impressive heights. This is a royal dish well worth the extra effort called for in its preparation, especially since it is rich in beta-carotene in the apricots, protease inhibitors in the nuts, and selenium in the eggs.

| | |
|---|---|
| 2 teaspoons butter | 3 tablespoons honey |
| ½ cup finely ground toasted almonds | ¼ teaspoon cream of tartar |
| 1 cup unsweetened apricot spread | Toasted slivered almonds for |
| 1 tablespoon lemon juice | garnish |
| 1 tablespoon arrowroot powder | Whipped cream for garnish |
| 4 eggs, separated | (optional) |

Preheat oven to 375 °F.

Butter bottom and sides of a 1½-quart soufflé dish and dust with ½ cup ground almonds.

Combine remaining ground almonds, apricot spread, lemon juice, arrowroot, egg yolks, and honey in blender or food processor and whiz until light and fluffy.

In another bowl, beat the egg whites until foamy. Add cream of tartar and continue beating until stiff peaks form. Fold about one-fourth of the egg whites into the apricot mixture and blend well. Gently fold in the remaining egg whites.

Pour batter into prepared soufflé dish and bake for 25 to 30 minutes. Remove from oven and decorate with slivered almonds and, on special occasions, with dollops of whipped cream. Serve immediately, since soufflé will fall rapidly.

**Yield:** 4 to 6 servings

---

Each of 4 servings provides 364 calories, 11 g protein, 7 g saturated fat, 7 g unsaturated fat, 54 mg sodium. Each of 6 servings provides 239 calories, 11 g protein, 5 g saturated fat, 5 g unsaturated fat, 36.6 mg sodium.

---

## CATSUP—A HEALTH FOOD?

Would you ever think of saying to your child, "Be sure to put some ketchup on your sandwich, honey. It's good for you"?

Hard to believe, isn't it? But, according to recent research, it's true.

We have long known that tomatoes contain lycopene, an important antioxidant. But a new study by Dr. Venket Rao of the University of Toronto and published in a recent issue of *Lipids* magazine reveals that *processed* tomato products like tomato sauce, tomato juice, and *catsup* provide about five times more lycopene than fresh tomatoes. Also it seems that heating the tomatoes makes it easier for the body to absorb the lycopene.

What tomato product is exposed to heat longer than any other? That's right—*catsup!* Therefore, when you and your children slather catsup on your hamburgers, you may be protecting the cells of your body from free radicals, which cause heart disease, cancer, and aging.

Another way to increase your consumption of catsup, according to Heinz, the country's largest producer of tomato products, especially catsup, is to serve a *love apple pie.*

"Love apple," you will recall, was the first name for "tomato." And yes, this pie is made with catsup. I was intrigued. So I made it. And, you know what? It was very good. Try it; you'll like it.

# Catsup-Apple Pie

This is my version of the love apple pie.

6 cups chopped or cut-up apples, preferably tart

⅓ cup catsup combined with 2 tablespoons lemon juice

½ teaspoon cinnamon

1 teaspoon grated orange rind (optional)

½ teaspoon freshly grated nutmeg

Prepared pie crust or about 6 crushed graham crackers

Graham cracker crumbs (optional)

Sesame seeds (optional)

Chopped sunflower seeds (optional)

Soy nuts (optional)

Chopped walnuts (optional)

Plain nonfat yogurt (optional)

Preheat oven to 350°F.

Combine the chopped apples with the catsup-lemon mixture. Stir in the cinnamon, orange rind (if desired), and nutmeg. Pile the mixture into the prepared pie crust if you're using it. Or pour it into a pie plate lined with crushed graham crackers.

Top with a mixture of graham cracker crumbs combined with sesame seeds, chopped sunflower seeds, soy nuts, and chopped walnuts.

Bake for about 25 minutes, or until the apples are softened and cooked through.

I like to serve it hot with a dollop of yogurt. Delicious!

*Yield:* 6 servings

Each serving provides 73 calories, 2.3 g protein, .6 g fat, 241 mg sodium.

# Prune Puree

This delicious puree will help you greatly reduce the fat in your favorite cake recipes.

1½ cups pitted prunes
6 tablespoons hot water

Combine both ingredients in food processor and puree until smooth.

If a recipe calls for 1 cup butter or oil, use ½ cup prune puree instead. You will greatly reduce the fat and the calories.

*Yield:* 1 cup

---

**Each ¼ cup provides 100 calories, 1 g protein, no fat, 5 mg sodium.**

---

# Fruit and Nut Bars

Soaking the almonds starts the sprouting process. The pineapple, dates, and coconut provide a medley of nutrients to delight your body and flavors to delight your taste buds.

½ cup almonds soaked in reserved pineapple juice for 2 hours or overnight
½ cup drained crushed pineapple, juice reserved
2 eggs
¼ cup molasses or honey

½ cup chopped dates
¼ cup unsweetened shredded coconut
½ cup whole wheat pastry flour
2 tablespoons soy powder or flour
2 tablespoons wheat germ

Preheat oven to 350 °F.

In mixing bowl, blender, or food processor, combine eggs, pineapple, almonds, molasses or honey, dates, and coconut, and mix well. Add the remaining dry ingredients and mix just enough to combine ingredients. Do not overmix.

Spread the mixture in a 9-inch-square baking dish lined with parchment paper or sprayed with nonstick cooking spray. Bake for 30 minutes, or until golden and firm. Cool slightly, then cut into 1½-inch squares.

*Yield:* 36 squares

---

Each square provides approximately 43 calories, 1.5 g protein, .3 g saturated fat, .5 g unsaturated fat, 3.9 mg sodium.

---

# Peanut Butter Balls

A confection you'll be happy to see children devour. It's loaded with vitamins, minerals, and antioxidants.

 ¾ cup peanut butter
 ¼ cup wheat germ
 2 tablespoons honey
 1 cup nonfat dry milk (spray dried)
 Toasted sesame seeds or finely chopped nuts

In a bowl or food processor, blend the peanut butter, wheat germ, honey, and milk powder. Form into balls and roll in sesame seeds or nuts.

*Yield:* 36 confections

**Each one provides approximately 15 calories, 1 g protein, trace saturated fat, 1.8 g unsaturated fat, 36 mg sodium.**

# Carob-Walnut Clusters

A crunchy, nutty treat, rich in strengthening nutrients, with a taste reminiscent of an old-time sweet shop.

| | |
|---|---|
| 2 tablespoons unsalted butter | 5 tablespoons carob powder |
| ¼ cup honey | ½ cup whole wheat pastry flour |
| 1 egg | 1½ cups coarsely chopped walnuts |
| 1½ teaspoons vanilla | |

In food processor, blender, or mixing bowl, mix together the butter, honey, egg, and vanilla. Add the carob powder and flour. Mix until ingredients are well combined, then stir in the walnuts.

Preheat oven to 325°F.

Drop the batter by teaspoonfuls onto a cookie sheet lined with parchment paper or sprayed with nonstick cooking spray. Bake for 15 minutes.

*Yield:* 36 enticing clusters

**Each cluster provides approximately 50 calories, 1 g protein, .6 g saturated fat, 2.5 g unsaturated fat, .6 mg sodium.**

# Apricot Chews

These crunchy gems are great for stashing in your purse or pockets for an on-hand battery charger. Each slice packs an antioxidant punch and also delivers a lot of fiber, a big dose of iron (about 1.3 mg in each slice), as well as vitamin A and calcium. Since these require no baking, kids can enjoy making a quick batch for get-togethers and pajama party snacking.

| | |
|---|---|
| 12 dried apricots | 2 tablespoons unsulphured molasses |
| Apple or orange juice, for soaking fruit | 2 tablespoons wheat germ |
| 6 dried figs | 2 tablespoons soy grits (textured vegetable protein) |
| ½ cup raisins | Unsweetened shredded coconut (optional) |
| ½ cup almonds | |
| ½ cup sunflower seeds | |

Soak apricots and figs in juice to cover for a few hours or overnight. Or, use only 2 tablespoons juice and microwave with the fruit on medium for 2 minutes.

Combine the softened apricots and figs, raisins, almonds, sunflower seeds, molasses, wheat germ, and soy grits in food processor or blender, and process until ingredients begin to coalesce.

On wax paper, form the batter into a sausagelike roll. Cover with coconut if you're using it. Refrigerate for a few hours, slice, and serve. Or divide into 24 portions and roll into balls.

*Yield:* 2 dozen ¹/₂-inch slices or walnut-size balls

---

**Each slice without coconut provides approximately 58 calories, 2.5 g protein, trace saturated fat, 1.5 g unsaturated fat, 3.5 mg sodium.**

---

# No-Fat Cookie Jar Hermits

A very healthy pleasure. The genistein provided by the soy flour adds its antioxidant potential to the vitamin E provided by the wheat germ, making these delicious hermits a boon to your body and a blessing to your taste buds.

1½ cups whole wheat pastry flour
¼ cup soy flour
½ cup wheat germ
½ teaspoon baking soda
½ teaspoon cinnamon
½ teaspoon freshly grated nutmeg
¼ teaspoon ground cloves
½ cup drained unsweetened apple
    or pear sauce

½ cup Sucanat
1 egg
¼ cup cold brewed coffee, regular or
    decaffeinated
1 cup seedless raisins
½ cup coarsely chopped walnuts

Preheat oven to 375°F.

Combine the flours, wheat germ, baking soda, cinnamon, nutmeg, and cloves in a bowl. Set aside.

In another bowl or a food processor, blend together the apple or pear sauce, the Sucanat, and the egg. Add the dry ingredients, one-third at a time alternately with the coffee. Stir in the raisins and nuts.

Drop by rounded teaspoonfuls about 2 inches apart on cookie sheets lined with parchment paper or sprayed with nonstick cooking spray. Bake for 10 minutes.

*Yield:* 24 cookies

Each cookie provides approximately 81 calories, 32.8 g protein, trace saturated fat, 1.3 g unsaturated fat, 5.5 mg sodium.

# Fantastic Fruity Bread Pudding

An ingenious way to transform day-old bread into a heavenly dish rich in hard-working antioxidants provided by the apricots, which are a superior source of vitamin A; prunes and raisins, which increase the vitamin A wallop and contribute many helpful minerals; and walnuts, a good source of the important omega-3 fatty acids so good for your heart and your brain.

| | |
|---|---|
| 3 eggs | 4 cups cubed bread |
| 3 tablespoons butter, softened | ½ cup oat bran |
| 1¾ cups skim milk | 3 tablespoons wheat germ |
| ¼ cup molasses | 12 dried apricots, slivered |
| 1 teaspoon vanilla | 12 prunes, slivered |
| 1½ teaspoons cinnamon | ½ cup raisins |
| ¼ teaspoon freshly grated nutmeg | ¼ cup chopped walnuts |

Preheat oven to 350°F.

In a mixing bowl or food processor, blend together the eggs, butter, milk, molasses, vanilla, cinnamon, and nutmeg.

In a buttered 13-by-9-by-2-inch baking dish, combine the cubed bread, oat bran, wheat germ, apricots, prunes, and raisins. Pour the egg mixture over the bread mixture. Top with chopped walnuts.

Bake for 45 to 50 minutes. Live it up—serve it with fresh raspberries and whipped cream.

## MICROWAVE METHOD

Follow above directions. Microcook on high in a covered dish for 8 minutes.

*Yield:* 10 servings

**Each serving provides 350 calories, 14 g protein, .3 g saturated fat, 16 g unsaturated fat, 48 g sodium.**

# Brazil Nut Cookies

Cooked parsnips give these delicious cookies their wonderful texture. A close relative of carrots, rich-in-fiber parsnips are now being investigated for compounds that may prevent the initiation of cancer.

The Brazil nuts are an excellent source of selenium, a powerful antioxidant.

| | |
|---|---|
| 1 egg | 1 cup whole wheat pastry flour, less |
| 2 tablespoons honey | 3 tablespoons |
| 2 tablespoons olive or canola oil | 3 tablespoons soy flour |
| 1 teaspoon vanilla | ½ cup wheat germ |
| 1 cup cooked parsnips, put through a sieve | 2 teaspoons baking powder |
| | ½ cup raisins |
| 1 cooked carrot, put through a sieve | 4 Brazil nuts, grated |

Preheat oven to 350°F.

In food processor, blender, or mixing bowl, combine egg, honey, oil, vanilla, and sieved parsnips and carrot. Blend until smooth and creamy.

In another bowl, combine flours, wheat germ, and baking powder. Add this mixture to the parsnip-carrot mixture and blend.

Stir in the nuts, raisins, and sesame seeds.

Drop the batter by tablespoonfuls on a cookie sheet lined with parchment paper or sprayed with nonstick cooking spray. Sprinkle Brazil nuts on each cookie. Bake for 12 to 15 minutes, or until lightly browned.

*Yield:* 3 dozen heavenly cookies

---

**Each cookie provides approximately 41 calories, 1 g protein, trace saturated fat, 2.7 g unsaturated fat, 3.5 mg sodium.**

# Carob Mint Pudding or Pie

A cool, refreshing creamy dessert you can enjoy without guilt. Carob tastes like chocolate but has no caffeine or theobromin, has no sugar but is naturally sweet, has much fewer calories, and is loaded with important antioxidant minerals. The tofu is a gold mine of genistein, a powerful antioxidant.

| | |
|---|---|
| 1½ pounds tofu | 1 egg |
| ½ cup light honey | ½ teaspoon cinnamon |
| ½ cup carob powder | ¼ teaspoon peppermint extract |
| 4 teaspoons vanilla extract | Unbaked pie shell |

## Topping

4 ounces tofu

1 tablespoon honey

1 teaspoon vanilla extract

Preheat oven to 400°F.

Combine all the ingredients except the pie shell in blender or food processor and process until very smooth. Enjoy as a pudding or pour into pie crust. Bake until crust begins to brown, about 15 minutes.

Cool and serve with tofu whipped cream. To make whipped cream, blend tofu with honey and vanilla in a food processor or beat well by hand.

*Yield:* 6 servings

**Each serving without the crust provides approximately 67 calories, .5 g protein, 10 g fat, 30 mg sodium.**

# Strawberry-Pineapple Compote

A dessert to freshen your body and your spirit. Pineapple in partnership with its enzyme, bromelain, aid digestion, help dissolve blood clots, and can help prevent osteoporosis because of a high content of bone-strengthening manganese. Strawberries, no slouch in the antioxidant parade, provide vitamins A, C, and some of the B vitamins. In the Far East, they are considered a warming food and are used medicinally to expel cold from the body's extremities.

> ¼ cup maple syrup
> 1½ tablespoons balsamic vinegar
> ½ teaspoon vanilla
> 2 cups thickly sliced strawberries
> 2 cups fresh or canned pineapple chunks

Stir together in a large bowl the maple syrup, vinegar, and vanilla.
Just before serving, combine the dressing with the fruit and mix gently.

*Yield:* 4 servings

---

**Each serving provides 120 calories, 1 g protein, 30 g carbohydrates, 1 g fat, no cholesterol, 5 mg sodium.**

---

# Banana Freeze

Bananas are nutritious and easily digested, which is why they appeal to young and old. One of my favorite ways to use bananas is in this creamy, luscious treat that is thicker than a milkshake but doesn't necessarily require a spoon. I like to add sunflower or pumpkin seeds, chopped almonds, Brazil nuts, walnuts, or lightly toasted soy nuts to the mixture.

3 or 4 ripe bananas, cut into chunks and frozen

Freeze the bananas for at least an hour. Remove from the freezer about 5 minutes before using.

Place the bananas in the food processor and whiz for 20 to 40 seconds, or until they form a thick silky substance similar to regular ice cream in consistency. Enjoy them plain or add the embellishment of your choice.

*Yield:* About 6 servings

---

**Each serving provides about 60 calories, no fat, no sodium.**

---

# Fruit Strudel

Strudel is typically reserved for special occasions. But don't wait to make it. Strudel makes any occasion great. The dough can be made with whole wheat pastry flour. It will taste very good but it will not be quite so "stretchy" as when made with unbleached white flour. If you choose to use the white, you can add vitamins and minerals by adding wheat germ to the filling, 1 tablespoon for each cup of flour. Sprinkle it on the rolled and stretched dough. The wheat germ is a source of vitamin E, a major antioxidant. The filling calls for a grated orange and a grated lemon, both sources of powerful antioxidants. Use the whole fruit, skin, pulp, everything except the seeds. Be sure to thoroughly scrub the fruit before grating. The apricots in the filling are a good source of beta-carotene.

## Filling

2 cups dried apricots, soaked in hot water for a few hours or overnight, or
    with only ¼ cup water in the microwave on medium for 2 minutes
¼ cup honey
1 whole lemon, grated and pitted
1 whole orange, grated and pitted

## Nut Mixture

1 cup crushed walnuts
½ teaspoon cinnamon
1 cup raisins, preferably golden
½ cup cake, cookie, or graham cracker crumbs
½ cup wheat germ
1 cup unsweetened shredded coconut

## Strudel Dough

1 egg
¼ cup vegetable oil (preferably canola)
6 tablespoons warm water
2 cups whole wheat pastry flour or unbleached white flour
A little more oil for drizzling over the dough
Ground walnuts (optional)

### TO PREPARE THE FILLING

Drain the water from the soaked apricots. (It makes a delicious fruit juice.)

In food processor, blender, or mixing bowl, blend together the soaked apricots, the honey, and half the grated lemon and orange. Reserve the other half for use with the nut mixture. The apricot mixture makes a great filling but you can substitute any good-quality fruit conserve, preferably unsweetened.

## TO MAKE THE NUT MIXTURE

Combine the walnuts, cinnamon, raisins, crumbs, wheat germ, coconut, and the reserved grated lemon and orange.

## TO MAKE THE DOUGH

In a medium-size bowl, beat the egg, add the oil and water, then the flour. Knead lightly until the dough is soft. Cover and set in a warm place for 1 hour.

Divide the dough in half. Place one half on a floured tablecloth and roll it out. Pull and stretch gently until the dough is so thin you can see through it.

After the dough has been stretched, spread half the nut mixture over the entire sheet. Drizzle a little oil over all. Spread one-fourth of the fruit mixture in a line across one end of the sheet about 3 inches from the edge. Fold this 3-inch edge over the fruit mixture; raise the tablecloth, and let the dough roll over itself to the halfway point. Follow the same procedure with the other half of the sheet.

Do the same with the second half of the dough and fruit and nut mixtures.

Place the rolls in a pan or on a cookie sheet lined with parchment paper or greased with a little oil. Brush the strudel with a bit of oil and top with the ground nuts, if desired. Let stand for about 15 minutes.

Preheat oven to 350°F.

Slice the strudel diagonally into 1-inch pieces, but do not cut all the way through. Bake for about 45 minutes. When cool, cut all the way through.

*Yield:* About 20 pieces

**Each piece provides approximately 119 calories, 29 g protein, trace saturated fat, 40 g unsaturated fat, 8 mg sodium.**

# Glossary of Antioxidants

With the discovery of the antioxidants in many of our foods in the latter segment of the twentieth century, a magic window was opened for all of us. We learned that we have the power in a sense to control our destiny, if we have the desire and the inclination to learn.

And that's why we wrote this book—*to bring you the knowledge that could save your life, and recipes to help you enjoy the process.* It combines the joy of cooking and the pleasures of the table with good sound health sense.

Where do you find these magical substances? They're not on the stock market. But you will find them in the fish market and growing on trees, vines, and bushes.

Here is a discussion of some of the major antioxidants in food.

**Allyl sulfides:** Found in garlic, onions, leeks, and chives, allyl sulfides facilitate the excretion of carcinogens.

**Beta-carotene:** It boosts immunity and is linked to preventing heart attacks, strokes, and cancer, especially lung cancer. It is found in dark green leafy vegetables like romaine, collard greens, kale, spinach, and broccoli and deep orange vegetables like sweet potatoes, carrots, pumpkin, mangos, and pink grapefruit. The darker the green, the more intense the orange, the more beta-carotene. It is not destroyed by cooking.

**Boron:** A mineral that can strengthen your bones and actually make you smarter by affecting the electrical activity of the brain. If you feel mentally sluggish and unable to cope, you may need more boron, which is provided by nuts, leafy vegetables, and fruits, especially grapes, peaches, apples, and pears, and by honey.

Not only does boron make you smarter, it helps prevent osteoporosis by minimizing the loss of calcium and magnesium from your bones. Aim for 3 milligrams a day, easily obtained from food and available from natural food stores in pill form.

**Co-enzyme Q10 (Ubiquinol):** A very good friend to your heart, Co-enzyme Q10 helps to remove the harmful effects of LDL (bad) cholesterol. It boosts the power of vitamin E, its partner in the promotion of heart health. Enjoy it bountifully in mackerel, sardines, soybeans, walnuts, pistachios, peanuts, and sesame seeds.

**Echinacea and goldenseal:** Echinacea, an herb that was used by some Indian tribes for many years to encourage wound healing, seems to bolster the immune system and may help to fight off colds. It seems to work best if taken at the very first sign of a cold and should be taken only when needed.

Goldenseal is a very effective partner for echinacea. It seems to help clear up infections and strengthen the mucous membranes in your nose and throat, thus reducing the agony of the common cold. Take them daily only when you need them, but for no longer than two weeks.

**Ellagic acid:** Found in grapes. It searches out carcinogens and prevents them from making damaging changes in DNA.

**Ginkgo biloba:** Keep forgetting where you put your eyeglasses? Let this powerful antioxidant help you to remember. According to James F. Balch, M.D., author of *Prescriptions for Nutritional Healing*, it even improves memory in Alzheimer's patients.

But this wonder-working antioxidant does much more. It boosts the ability of vitamins C and E to defend the immune system. It improves peripheral and cerebral circulation. Dr. Balch recommends it for tinnitus, asthma, heart, and kidney disorders and for glucose utilization. To get the most from this antioxidant, you need 60 to 80 milligrams three times a day.

**Glutathione:** It knocks out cancer by deactivating the substances that trigger cancer. The best sources are avocados, asparagus, watermelon, grapefruit, okra, white potatoes, squash, and cauliflower. Canned and processed foods have much less glutathione activity than the fresh or frozen.

**Grape seed extract:** Who among us does not need this miraculous substance that goes to bat for the blood vessels on which our very lives depend? Just think. It helps your blood vessels carry life-saving oxygen to prevent damage to your heart, to your brain to help guard against stroke, and to guard against varicose veins, bleeding gums, and edema.

If you can find grapes with their seeds intact, it wouldn't hurt at all to chew those seeds. But you don't have to in order to benefit from their wondrous effects. To the rescue comes the French Connection, a lifesaving combination of grape seeds and pine bark, called *pycnogenol.*

The strong antioxidant activity of pycnogenol has been used successfully to relieve eye strain, to treat retinopathy, and to delay progression of macular degeneration. The usual dose is 100 to 150 milligrams daily.

**Indoles:** By detoxifying free radicals, indoles help to prevent colon and breast cancer and are provided by the cruciferous family, which includes cabbage, cress, cauliflower, broccoli, Brussels sprouts, kale, kohlrabi, turnips, and radishes. If you cook these vegetables, be sure to save the cooking water. That's where they leave half their indoles.

**Limonene:** Found in citrus fruits, it boosts enzymes that wipe out cancer-causing substances.

**Lycopene:** A powerful antioxidant that throws a monkey wrench into devastating chain reactions of destructive free radical molecules. The tomato family is the best source.

It is also found in watermelon and in apricots.

It is not destroyed by cooking. In fact cooking releases more of the wonder-working lycopene. It has been found that the longer tomatoes are cooked, the more lycopene is released for active duty. That means that tomato sauce, tomato paste, and even the staple catsup are valuable sources of wonder-working lycopene, which has been linked to lower rates of pancreatic and cervical cancers.

**Protease Inhibitors:** Protease inhibitors are potent bodyguards. They squelch cancer by interfering with the activity of enzymes called proteases, which can promote cancer. Protease inhibitors are very special protectors because they have the rare power to prevent normal cells from pursuing the disastrous road to malignancy even after the cancerous course has been initiated, even if it is already in the early stages.

These protective agents are found in soybeans, chick peas, lima beans, kidney beans, fava beans, peas, lentils, tofu, and whole grains (especially flax and oats), all kinds of nuts and seeds, white potatoes, sweet potatoes, and sweet corn.

**Quercetin:** A bioflavonoid and very potent antioxidant, quercetin stops trouble before it begins by knocking out several cancer-causing agents and inhibiting enzymes that encourage the growth of tumors. It is found in red and yellow onions, shallots, red grapes, and broccoli. Happily, it is not destroyed by cooking or freezing.

**Selenium:** Works in partnership with vitamin E, fights viral infections, even HIV, the virus which causes AIDS. It also helps protect the eyes from cataracts and the heart from muscle damage.

The soil on which most of our produce is grown is now deficient in this important mineral, which is plentiful in Brazil. And that's why Brazil nuts are an excellent source. It takes only one or two nuts to meet the daily value of 70 micrograms.

**Vitamins A, C, and E:** Jean Carper reports in her book, *Food: Your Miracle Medicine* that a twelve-year study of about 3,000 men in Switzerland revealed that those with low blood levels of carotene and vitamin A were more apt to die of all types of cancer, especially lung cancer. Low blood levels of vitamin C predicted death from stomach and gastrointestinal cancer.

Vitamin A plays many important roles. It is essential for healthy skin and mucous membranes and to the production of visual purple, which guards against night blindness. And that's not all. It boosts your immunity, especially against colds and other respiratory ailments.

Vitamin A is fat soluble and occurs in two forms: preformed vitamin A and provitamin A. Preformed vitamin A is a compound called retinol and occurs in foods of animal origin such as butter, eggs, milk, and liver.

Beta-carotene or provitamin A is one of 600 carotenoids found in dark green leafy vegetables and in yellow and orange fruits and vegetables. Good food sources are apricots, broccoli, carrots, cantalope, mangoes, papaya, peaches, spinach, yellow squash, sweet potatoes, and pumpkin.

When vitamin E was first discovered in 1920, it was called tocopherol, which in Greek means "to bring forth children."

It does not affect your ability to conceive. It does enhance your ability to carry to term. I had my first experience with the magical power of vitamin E back in 1940 when I experienced a miscarriage. Instead of putting me on the drug that was then being touted to prevent miscarriage and which later was found to cause cancer in the genitals of the female children then conceived, my very knowledgeable physician put me on vitamin E, which then enabled me to carry all four of my children to term.

We have made much progress, conducted many scientific studies, and now realize that vitamin E is a potent antioxidant. It protects the fatty acids in our cells from free radical damage that has been linked to both cancer and heart disease.

Vitamin E is acknowledged as a leading protector of the arteries and the heart. It also helps ease leg cramps and restless leg syndrome.

Vitamin E works in partnership with selenium. To get enough vitamin E and selenium, take the two together and you will greatly enhance the potency of both. Some food sources of vitamin E are whole grains, wheat germ, brown rice, sweet potatoes, vegetable oils, avocadoes, oats, peanuts, almonds, walnuts, and other nuts.

# Index

**JANE KINDERLEHRER**, the author of Newmarket's classic "Smart Food" cookbook series, was senior editor and food editor of *Prevention* magazine and a regular *New York Times* columnist. She is also the author of *Confessions of a Sneaky Organic Cook, How to Feel Younger Longer, The Art of Cooking with Love and Wheat Germ,* and *Cooking Kosher the New Way.*

**DANIEL A. KINDERLEHRER, M.D.,** is a practicing physician in Danvers, Massachusetts, and a clinical instructor at Tufts Medical School. Dr. Kinderlehrer evaluates and treats patients from a holistic perspective, with particular interests in diet and nutrition; food and environmental sensitivities; lifestyle, emotional, and stress factors; and spiritual attunement. He lectures widely and has been a regular presenter at the Omega Institute in Rhinebeck, New York, and Interface in Boston, Massachusetts. He has three children and lives in Santa Fe, New Mexico.

**Ask for these Jane Kinderlehrer titles at your local bookstore or order today.**

Use this coupon or write to Newmarket Press, 18 East 48th Street, New York, NY 10017 (212) 832-3575.

Please send me:

### The Smart Baking Cookbook—Muffins, Cookies, Biscuits, and Breads

More than 180 recipes for heavenly, healthful muffins, cookies, biscuits, breads, and toppings—high in fiber and protein and low in fat, sodium, and cholesterol. Plus, instructions on wheat-, sugar-, and dairy-free baking.

"Kinderlehrer knows how to strike a balance between taste and nutrition that will have diners clamoring for more." —*Publishers Weekly*

___ $16.95, paperback, 304 pages (ISBN 978-1-55704-522-5)
___ $21.95, hardcover, 304 pages (ISBN 978-1-55704-281-1)

### The Smart Chicken & Fish Cookbook—Over 200 Delicious and Nutritious Recipes for Main Courses, Soups, and Salads

Delectable fish and fowl recipes for main courses, soups, and salads—all high-fiber, low-fat, low- or no-sugar, low sodium, and low cholesterol.

"[Kinderlehrer] not only steers you to delicious and nutritious eating, but also gives you the facts you need to be informed."

*—The International Cookbook Revue*

___ $16.95, paperback, 320 pages (ISBN 978-1-55704-544-7)

---

For postage and handling, add $5.00 for the first book, plus $1.50 for each additional book. Prices and availability subject to change. (New York residents, please add applicable state and local taxes.)

I enclose a check or money order, payable to Newmarket Press, in the amount of $_____.

Name _____

Address _____

City/State/Zip _____

Clubs, firms, and other organizations may qualify for special discounts when ordering quantities of these titles. For more information, please call or write Newmarket Press, Special Sales Department, 18 East 48th Street, New York, NY 10017; call (212) 832-3575 or (800) 669-3903; fax (212) 832-3629; or e-mail info@newmarketpress.com.

**www.newmarketpress.com**

Antioxidant 6/07